Effective Health Care Management

An evaluative approach

Colin Palfrey
School of Health Science,
University of Wales Swansea

Paul Thomas
University of Wales Swansea & University of Glamorgan, Wales

Ceri Phillips
School of Health Science,
University of Wales Swansea

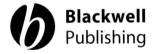
Blackwell
Publishing

© 2004 C. Palfrey, P. Thomas & C. Phillips

Blackwell Publishing Ltd
Editorial offices:
Blackwell Publishing Ltd, 9600 Garsington
Road, Oxford OX4 2DQ, UK
 Tel: +44 (0)1865 776868
Blackwell Publishing Inc., 350 Main Street,
Malden, MA 02148-5020, USA
 Tel: +1 781 388 8250
Blackwell Publishing Asia Pty Ltd, 550
Swanston Street, Carlton, Victoria 3053,
Australia
 Tel: +61 (0)3 8359 1011

First published 2004 by Blackwell Publishing Ltd

Library of Congress Cataloging-in-Publication
Data
Palfrey, Colin, 1939–
 Effective health care management : an
evaluative approach / Colin Palfrey, Paul
Thomas, Ceri Phillips. – 1st ed.
  p. ; cm.
 Includes bibliographical references
and index.
 ISBN 1-4051-1161-5 (pbk. : alk. paper)
 1. Health services administration.
2. Medical care – Evaluation.
 [DNLM: 1. Health Services
Administration – standards. 2. Efficiency,
Organizational. 3. Health Care Evaluation
Mechanisms – organization &
administration. 4. Quality Assurance,
Health Care – organization &
administration. W 84.1 P159e 2004]
 I. Thomas, Paul (Paul Randal), 1945–
 II. Phillips, Ceri. III. Title.
RA394.P287 2004
362.1′068–dc22   2003022945

ISBN 1-4051-1161-5

A catalogue record for this title is available
from the British Library

Set in 12/14pt Times
by Graphicraft Limited, Hong Kong
Printed and bound in India
by Replika Press Pvt. Ltd, Kundli 131028

The publisher's policy is to use permanent
paper from mills that operate a sustainable
forestry policy, and which has been
manufactured from pulp processed using
acid-free and elementary chlorine-free
practices. Furthermore, the publisher ensures
that the text paper and cover board used have
met acceptable environmental accreditation
standards.

For further information on
Blackwell Publishing, visit our website:
www.blackwellpublishing.com

Effective Health Care Management

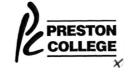
William Tuson
Library & Learning Centre
Tel: 01772 225310

PRESTON
COLLEGE

Please return or renew on or before the date shown below.
Fines will be charged on overdue items.

Contents

Dedication

We wish to dedicate this book to our former colleague and friend, David Edwards. He was, indeed, a good chap.

Preface

Many books have been written on management in health care systems. What is different about this one? It is not a 'how to do it' book for health care managers though we do explore a number of issues which are important for them.

Compared with other books this one focuses much more explicitly on 'evaluation' in health care management. A wide range of stakeholders make judgements about what the public's principal health care needs are, about what the health care system should be achieving, about the various means by which those objectives should be achieved, about how health care policies should be implemented and about how health care policies and the performance of the system should be evaluated. Health care managers often work in an ambiguous context of central-local decision making, probably more so than managers in other public sector organisations. They, therefore, require sensitivity to different perspectives on how and where resources should be targeted.

This book directly addresses these evaluative processes and argues that there will inevitably be conflicting views among the various stakeholders – including health care professionals – for example doctors, nurses and the professions allied to medicine, health care managers; state institutions such as the Commission for Healthcare Audit and Inspection and the National Institute for Clinical Excellence; politicians; recipients of specific services; pressure groups; the mass media; and the public at large.

Some stakeholders may see efficiency as the main evaluative criterion to be used in making judgements about the health care system. Others may insist that effectiveness is more important than efficiency. Yet others will espouse the

importance of equity or equality, and so forth. These conflicting priorities exemplify the inherently partisan nature of
health care management. In evaluating the performance of
the health care system judgements have to be made about
what data are to be collected, about how the data are to be
collected and by whom and from whom, about the criteria –
and their weighting – to be used in translating the data into
useful information and about how the results of the evaluation should be fed back into the next phase of the policy
process.

Given that these questions are often tackled in different
ways by different stakeholders we should not be surprised
that performance indicators, government targets, league
tables and star ratings generate strong feelings among the
stakeholders. In this sense the health care system is no different from many other public services, such as education and
crime reduction policies. But the health care system does seem
to generate particularly strong feelings and does seem to go
through major reorganisations more frequently than other
services. Amongst all these changes are there any relatively
stable principles which health care managers and others can
cling to? One answer to this question might be the importance of being explicit about the criteria by which health care
policies and performance may be evaluated. Particular
approaches to evaluation – such as league tables and moun-
tains of government imposed detailed targets – may wax and
wane, but the need to be clear about the ways in which evaluative criteria in the health care system may be used – by
managers and others – is likely to remain an important issue
as an evaluative culture increasingly takes hold. It is to this
issue that this book is addressed.

Abbreviations

BAMM	British Association of Medical Managers
BMC	BioMed Central
BV	best value
BVPI	best value performance indicator
BVPP	best value performance plan
BVR	best value review
CCT	compulsory competitive tendering
CEO	chief executive officer
CHAI	Commission for Healthcare Audit and Inspection
CHD	coronary heart disease
CHI	Commission for Health Improvement
CHMR	Center for Health Management Research
CPA	comprehensive performance assessment
CPD	continuing professional development
EBC	evidence-based care
EBHC	evidence-based health care
EBM	evidence-based medicine
EBO	evidence-based organisation
EPOC	effective practice and organisation of care
FGE	fourth-generation evaluation
GI	gastro-intestinal
GORD	gastro-oesophageal reflux disease
HA	health authority
HCM	health care management
HTA	health technology assessment
IHM	Institute of Health Care Management
IHSM	Institute of Health Service Managers
IPR	individual performance review
LA	local authority

MCI	management charter initiative
NAO	National Audit Office
NICE	National Institute for Clinical Excellence
NSAID	non-steroidal anti-inflammatory drug
NSF	National Service Framework
PAC	Public Accounts Committee
PCG	primary care group
PCT	primary care trust
PDP	personal development plan
PI	performance indicators
PM	performance management
PONV	post-operative nausea and vomiting
PPIs	proton pump inhibitors
PSA	public service agreement
QALY	quality-adjusted life year
RHA	regional health authorities
RP	reflective practice
SA	staff appraisal
SMART	specific, measurable, achievable, relevant/ realistic timed
TQM	total quality management

Chapter 1
Introduction

Our argument in this book is that evaluation is a crucial, indeed an inevitable and inherent part of the work of health care professionals and health service managers. Our aim is to help health professionals and managers within health care systems to develop their critical understanding of the issues and problems involved in evaluating the performance of those systems and to help readers to develop their ability to undertake robust evaluations of the services that they, and others, provide. Whether evaluations are being undertaken by the professionals and managers themselves or by others – such as external agencies – we believe it is important for those working within health care systems to be aware of what evaluation involves, why and how it is done and to be able to contribute to useful evaluations in a key part of the public services.

'Evaluation' is concerned with 'judging merit against some yardstick' (Phillips *et al.*, 1994, p. 1) and it is important to recognise that most evaluations are in fact not called 'evaluations'. They are often described as reviews, appraisals, assessments, audits, inspections, accreditations or as some other term which encompasses the notion of making judgements. Professionals and managers are thus involved in evaluations on a day to day basis. They range from the informal and intuitive, for example managers asking themselves whether things are going well, to the formal and explicit, for example an inspection by the Audit Commission.

Early thoughts about evaluative criteria

There are many criteria available when undertaking evaluations and what follows is a list (in no particular order) of those suggested by Maxwell (1984) as indicators of 'quality' in health care:

- effectiveness
- efficiency
- equity
- appropriateness
- acceptability
- accessibility

In practice, the use of these criteria would require managers and health care professionals to address the following questions.

Effectiveness   Do we have an explicit set of goals and objectives? To what extent are we achieving our goals and objectives? How can we improve the extent to which we are achieving our goals and objectives?

Efficiency   Do we know what benefits are being provided for the intended beneficiaries of our services? What goods and services are being provided? What impact are these having on the health of our patients and the community generally? What is the cost of delivering these benefits? How can we increase the ratio of the benefits to the costs?

Equity   Do we have a clear idea of the health needs of our patients and of the community generally? Do we deliver health care according to those needs? For example, do we provide equal care to those with the same needs? Do we differentiate appropriately? For example, do we provide more care for those in greater need? Is our service delivery seen by people as 'fair'?

Appropriateness   Is the care we are giving suitable for the health care needs of people? How can we ensure that our services remain relevant to what people need? (That is, are they based on a needs analysis rather than on historical patterns?)

Acceptability   To what extent do people approve of what we are doing and the ways in which we are providing services? How happy are patients and their families with our services? Do we take appropriate notice of the views of patients' forums and other representative groups? How satisfied is the local community with what we are doing?

Accessibility   To what extent do people have easy access to our services? How can we reduce inpatient and outpatient waiting times? Do we deliver services in accessible locations? Is physical access easy for disabled people? Is it easy for people to find their way around the system? Do people have easy access to the information they need?

We find Maxwell's list of criteria for evaluating the quality of services a useful one, but in some circumstances it is limited in its range. Later in this book, in Chapter 4, we propose to widen its scope to include additional criteria.

A conceptual framework

The conceptual framework which we find most useful for thinking about evaluation is a modified version of the well established 'systems model' (Easton, 1965). As Hill has pointed out (1997, pp. 20–22), the systems model has been the subject of criticism from a variety of sources, but as long as due attention is paid to the micro and macro political issues, it remains a useful framework. Our elaboration on the Easton model is illustrated in Figure 1.1.

The large bold-line rectangle (containing the various smaller text boxes) represents a 'system'. This could be an organisation, for example a hospital, an NHS trust, a primary care trust (a local health board in Wales or an NHS board in Scotland); a part of an organisation, for example a department, a directorate or a hospital ward; or a combination of organisations, for example a primary care trust seeking to work in partnership with social service agencies, or even the whole of the NHS.

The 'inputs' (top left of the diagram) represent anything which enters the system and thus include finance and information (for example the results of an evaluation, entering from

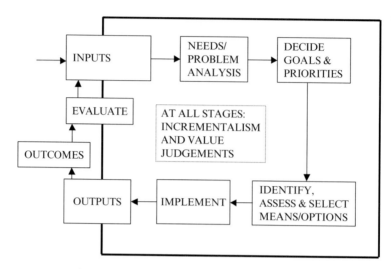

Figure 1.1   Modified systems model (modification of Thomas, 1988)

the box beneath the input box in the diagram, or information about what people's health care needs are, such as demands from gatekeepers like general practitioners, or the results of health surveys). They also include political influences from government and parliament, for example policy documents and legislation, and economic, social and technological pressures and influences from a wide variety of sources.

Within the system, staff are expected to collect and analyse information as to what the health care needs of people are (or are likely to be). Armed with this information, decisions then need to be made about what needs to be achieved (goals and objectives on the top right of the diagram) in order to meet the identified needs. Decisions also need to be made (and this is commonly one of the most difficult parts of the process) about what the priorities are, given that it is unlikely that all needs can be met.

To the extent that decision makers seek to make their decisions *rationally* (Simon, 1957) they will then seek alternative ways of achieving the agreed goals and objectives and will evaluate each method in order to decide on the *best* way forward (bottom right of diagram). *Best* here might mean the most efficient, most effective, most equitable, etc. depending on what criteria are considered most appropriate for making the necessary judgements. Such judgements can be very difficult, as can be seen, for example, in the following clinical management case study.

Case study on NSAIDS (based on Phillips, 2002)

There are about 24 million prescriptions written for non-steroidal anti-inflammatory drugs (NSAIDs) per year in the UK, with around 50% given to patients aged over 60, and 15% of the elderly population taking an NSAID at any one point in time.

The *benefits* of NSAIDS
They are important in the control of both acute and chronic pain and have also been shown to be effective in patients with moderate to severe post-operative pain. The benefits of aspirin, for example, in preventing cardiovascular events are well known, while there is also evidence for its effectiveness in reducing the incidence of and mortality from colon cancer.

The *risks* and their *avoidance*
However, NSAIDs are important causes of upper gastro-intestinal (GI) ulceration and dyspeptic symptoms, and in order to reduce risk acid-suppressing medication is often co-prescribed, with proton pump inhibitors (PPIs) increasingly the drug of choice. It is also known that PPIs are highly effective but relatively expensive gastro-protective agents in the healing and maintenance of NSAID induced ulcers. Therefore, a major dilemma confronts those who have to determine patient treatment regimens. An effective treatment is available but because of associated risks there are additional costs which need to be taken into consideration, against the background of limited resources and pressures to contain budgets, to prescribe generically and at the lowest possible cost.

What *decision*?
The problem of selecting the 'best' option is clearly not always a simple process.

The plans which emerge from these processes will be expected to be implemented in order to deliver goods and services to the health system's intended beneficiaries – either narrowly defined as the direct recipient of a particular health care intervention/treatment or defined broadly (as in the case of public health interventions such as health and safety policies or air pollution control) as the population generally.

All being well, these 'outputs' (goods and services – shown in the bottom left of the diagram) will then have outcomes, which are intended to have a positive impact on people's health. These outcomes or impacts are the most important things to evaluate (to judge the effect of what the services have brought about). Unfortunately they are also the most difficult elements to evaluate, partly because it is difficult to assess some aspects of health (especially in relation to quality of life) and partly because of the problem of causality. What we mean by this is that it is commonly difficult to be sure that a particular health policy has caused what *appears* to be the outcome of that policy. This is particularly the case with health and ill health, the determining factors of which are many and varied. An improvement in life expectancy in a particular population might be brought about by improvements in diet, life style, behavioural patterns, economic conditions, physical environmental conditions, medical interventions or various combinations of these. Trying to establish the relative contributions of the various factors to health 'outcomes' is notoriously problematic.

One possible way around this problem was shown in an evaluation of a health promotion programme designed to reduce smoking prevalence. Given that it was impossible to assess the specific contribution of the programme (and exclude other factors), a range of 'impact percentages' were used and the analysis provided an indication of the benefits accruing if the programme was responsible for between 10% and 100% of the decline in smoking achieved (Phillips & Prowle, 1993).

It is one of the tasks of managers and professionals when they (or others) are evaluating outcomes to try to judge whether what appears to be the impact of a policy really is causally connected to the policy in question. The results of such evaluations are then expected to be fed back into the system as an input to further developments in policy, thus returning us to the top left of the diagram once again.

It should be noticed that evaluation occurs twice in this process. It occurs when making judgements about what policies to adopt (the assessing and selecting options on the right hand side of the diagram) and again after the 'implementation' stage in order to judge what effects the policy has had.

However, to see the model as a series of stages is rather misconceived, and the boxes in the diagram are linked with sequential arrows more in the spirit of prescription than an accurate description of how policy processes work in practice. In reality the process is often more iterative than linear, for example a policy might need to be revisited and possibly amended during the implementation stage. An example of this is the way in which *Health of the Nation* targets (Department of Health, 1992) were later modified, for instance, to reflect the impact of deprivation on health (Baggott, 1998, p. 294).

It is important to recognise the significance of the box in the middle of the diagram (incrementalism and value judgements). This recognises some of the major limitations of the rational model which some other elements of our system model implies. As Lindblom argued (1959, 1979) political processes (in the partisan rather than party sense) are likely to influence all aspects of policy processes. It would be a very strange world if we all agreed with each other about everything all the time. Conflicts of opinion and of interests are ubiquitous and we need to recognise that there are likely to be differences of opinion and of values within the various stages of the policy process – needs assessment, goal setting, preferences about how to achieve the goals, implementation and evaluation. Policies and decisions, and non-decisions (Bachrach & Baratz, 1963) are likely to be the result, partly at least, of those with competing views negotiating for their preferred options and views. These preferences and perceptions will be affected by people's value judgements, attitudes and emotions (Mark, 2001; Vince, 2001).

Our model is, therefore, very different from the view of a system as a rational and objective framework. In our framework, what some people see as rational and linear processes are sandwiched between political processes at three levels:

- *macro level*, with political and other influences entering the system as inputs (top left hand corner of the Figure 1.1) from governments, interest groups, and others at *national* and *international* levels
- *meso level*, including normal *organisational* processes (for example at the level of primary care trusts and NHS trusts)
- *micro level*, including the working out of conflicts (both latent and real) at the level of *individual* professionals and managers

We believe the systems model, at least in its modified form, is an extremely useful framework for analysing and evaluating policy processes within health care systems. The value of the model, despite its limitations, is still widely recognised. Senge (1990) argues that the systems model is a powerful device for enabling people to understand how the various elements in a system and its sub-systems depend on each other, thus enabling us to see the 'big picture'.

These interrelationships and interdependencies are particularly important in the case of services which are expected to be planned and delivered by several organisations working in 'joined-up' collaborative partnerships. Calls for such joint working are not new (Booth, 1981) and despite the problems of achieving effective inter-organisational collaboration (Wistow, 1982; Challis *et al.*, 1988; Palfrey *et al.*, 1991; Webb, 1991; Huxham, 1996) the calls remain a high priority (Hudson *et al.*, 1999; Audit Commission, 2002; National Assembly for Wales, 2001). Health care needs are rarely compartmentalised according to convenient organisational boundaries.

An example of the continuing emphasis on the need for a systems view is the Audit Commission's 2002 report

Integrating services for older people: building a whole system approach in England in which the Commission strongly argues for a systems view in order to move from a fragmented approach to the planning and delivery of services to one in which a more strategic and collaborative model is developed. The version of the systems model which we have adopted (Figure 1.1) is helpful in relation to:

- helping people to focus on important (both 'hard' and 'soft') elements of the policy process, such as the setting of objectives in relation to the needs of the intended beneficiaries of health care systems
- encouraging a rational approach (despite the limitations of rational models) to decision making, including the evaluation of options and of outputs and outcomes
- acknowledging that there are important extra-rational elements to decision making, such as self-interest, ideological commitments, attitudes, perceptions and other political variables (Checkland, 1981)

Evaluation: the issues

Health care professionals and managers are involved in making judgements every day of their working lives. Sometimes these judgements/evaluations are explicit and systematic as in systematic reviews, the promotion of evidence-based practice and the use of 'best value' or 'value for money' thinking, and sometimes more intuitive and informal, as when people ask themselves whether things are going well. However, there are a number of long-standing evaluation issues, dilemmas and debates which confront people working in health care systems. One of these is the question of which criteria should be used in undertaking the evaluations.

Other issues include what may be seen as the unnecessary battles between people in ontological and epistemological debates (that is debates about the nature of things and about what counts as valid knowledge about them) concerning *positivism* and *interpretive* approaches to data collection and analysis. Put briefly, and therefore crudely, given the philosophical and complex nature of the issue, positivists believe that it is desirable and possible to maintain a clear distinction between a researcher (or 'evaluator') and that which is being researched (or in the case of evaluation, the 'evaluand'). Positivists argue that the evaluator can thus be 'objective' and can learn about something in a way that is quite independent of the researcher/evaluator – what one learns only concerns the evaluand and nothing is revealed about the evaluator.

Those who lean more towards the interpretive paradigm argue that absolute objectivity is impossible and that it is important to recognise the inevitable and inescapable element of subjectivity which will always be involved when people are seeking to learn about something. This element of subjectivity can show itself in many ways. In evaluating a policy or a service, the subjectivity is present in the selection of the criteria to be used in the evaluation, the interpretation of the criteria and the weighting of them. Furthermore, subjectivity is likely to be present not only for individuals but also on a collective level as when, for example, interest groups have commitments (ideological or pragmatic) to particular values, goals or specific projects, such as resisting the closure of a local hospital.

Davies & Nutley have pointed out (2000, p. 59) that one of the weaknesses of much research in health care has been:

> an obsession with discovering aggregate effects leading to a narrow focus on a positivistic paradigm (randomised control trials) to the relative exclusion of other methodological approaches (especially qualitative methods).

A helpful discussion of what some people see as the rival paradigms can be found in Burrell & Morgan (1979) and the alternative ontological and epistemological positions are summarised in Clarke (1999, pp. 38–41), but we do not necessarily accept that the paradigms need to be regarded as 'rivals'. Rather we agree with Davies (2000, p. 309) who suggests that 'evidence-based policy and practice requires both types of research and needs to foster an intellectual environment in which the complementary nature of qualitative and quantitative research can flourish'.

Another consideration, as we have suggested, is the variety of mechanisms available to undertake evaluations. They include:

- inspectorial approaches, such as inspections by the Audit Commission
- audits, either of clinical practice or financial management
- academic research
- management consultancy projects
- government-sponsored approaches, for example data relating to performance indicators and league tables
- accreditations, such as applications relating to Investors in People, Chartermark, ISO 9000 or the Business Excellence Model (of the European Foundation for Quality Management)
- managers monitoring the progress of work

In all of these approaches there are people making judgements against explicit criteria. The relationship between the various mechanisms and the criteria that each commonly incorporates has been examined elsewhere (Thomas & Palfrey, 1996) and will be further discussed in Chapter 3.

Another issue that managers and professionals need to be aware of is the distinction between criterion referenced and norm referenced evaluations. In the case of the former, a service, organisation or policy is judged according to the extent to which it has performed in relation to the criterion in question. For example, if an organisation (or part of an organisation, or an individual professional or manager) has achieved its explicit objectives then it can reasonably claim that it has done well in relation to the criterion of 'effectiveness'.

However, in the case of norm referenced evaluations, judgements are made in terms of how well or badly the organisation or service has done in relation to other comparable organisations. An obvious example of this is the use of league tables in which organisations, such as hospitals or even individual surgeons, are judged relative to others. The results of norm referencing need to be treated carefully. For example, it might be that survival rates following a particular kind of operation are significantly poorer for one surgeon than another; but this might be simply because the 'poorer' surgeon has a good reputation for dealing with difficult cases and has a greater number of such complex cases referred to him or her. Thus the relatively poor position in a league table might well be misleading. A more general problem with league tables and other forms of norm referencing is that the resultant data only tells us about performance relative to other organisations or individuals. The data says nothing about the performance against other explicit criteria.

A further distinction worth making is that between formative and summative assessments. This is analogous to the difference between concurrent and retrospective evaluations. The former is a kind of continuous monitoring from which one can learn to improve ongoing performance. The latter is done at a later stage when one looks back and says 'how did we do?' as opposed to 'how are we doing?'. Both forms are useful in their place, with formative assessments being particularly valuable when there is a need for 'continuous feedback during the course of a programme or project' (Phillips *et al.*, 1994, p. 2). The two forms can be used in conjunction with each other.

A similar, but different, distinction is that between process evaluations and output or outcome evaluations. In the former, the purpose is to evaluate the ways in which agreed work is being implemented (see the 'implement' box in Figure 1.1), whereas in the latter, judgements will be made about the goods and services which have been delivered and/or the impact that those outputs have had on the target population. As we noted earlier, the outcomes are the most important aspect to evaluate but also the most difficult.

Whatever kind of evaluation is carried out it is important for decision makers to be able to use the evaluation results so that policies and services may be improved in the light of what has been learned. As Rossi & Freeman have argued, 'the worth of evaluations must be judged by their utility' (1993, p. 443). An excellent summary of the issues involved in the utilisation of evaluation results is provided in Clarke (1999, pp. 173–85).

Who are the stakeholders in evaluation? Elsewhere (Thomas & Palfrey, 1996) we have argued that there are three main groups of stakeholders. These are:

- those who commission the services which are to be evaluated
- the intended beneficiaries of the services, both direct and indirect
- those who provide the services, either directly or indirectly; that is the (health care) professionals, the managers and the politicians

When services are being evaluated the views and interests of all these groups should be taken into account. In fact, with a collaborative approach, evaluations should be undertaken in such a way that a range of data needs to be collected and analysed and the data should be collected in a variety of appropriate methods and from a variety of sources. This is the core of 'pluralistic evaluation', an idea which was developed effectively by Smith & Cantley (1985) who evaluated hospital services from the points of view of patients, patients' relatives, health care professionals, managers, and others. One of the great benefits of pluralistic evaluation is that the service can be judged from several different perspectives, an important part of achieving a 'balanced' picture of the service, though this leaves unanswered the question of whose perspective is the most important and whose opinion should be given most weight. Should it be the patients, the taxpayer, the health care professionals and managers, the politicians, the community at large, some combination of these and/or others? We return to the issue of pluralistic evaluation in Chapter 3.

Fourth-generation evaluation

Guba & Lincoln (1989) have also considered the importance of 'value pluralism' in evaluations. For Guba & Lincoln the first generation of evaluation began to form early in the twentieth century and was characterised as 'technical', with the evaluator's role being that of technician. In this phase, evaluation meant little more than *measurement*; for example determining the status of individual pupils with respect to norms that had been established for certain standardised tests. Second-generation evaluation was characterised by *descriptions* of patterns and strengths and weaknesses with respect to certain stated objectives. Third-generation evaluation (which emerged in the mid-1960s) involved *judgements*. This approach required the objectives themselves to be treated as problematic (as opposed to accepting them as 'given'). Goals, no less than performance, were to be subject to evaluation. Fourth-generation evaluation, commonly referred to as *responsive*, takes as its point of focus not objectives, decisions or effects etc., but the claims, concerns and issues of various *stakeholders* and audiences. Such audiences include agents (developers, funders, implementers), beneficiaries (e.g. target groups) and victims (e.g. excluded target groups, potential beneficiaries of opportunities forgone). An important element in this generation is *value-pluralism*. Here the evaluator cannot ethically undertake to render judgements. What he or she has to do is to act as mediator in a negotiation process. The theme of negotiation is the hallmark of fourth-generation evaluation.

According to Guba & Lincoln (1989) the fundamental features of fourth-generation evaluation (FGE) are:

(1) *Value-pluralism*   FGE is the first kind of evaluation that explicitly recognises the possibility, indeed the appropriateness, of value-pluralism. Earlier generations tended to assume value-consensus but conflict is seen as normal in FGE. It would, therefore, not be enough merely to accept and apply a particular set of criteria for evaluation (for example the three Es of effectiveness, efficiency and economy, the 'value for money' concept initiated by the Audit Commission in the 1980s) without contesting the criteria from the viewpoint of other stakeholders.

(2) *The important role of stakeholder constructions*   FGE is rooted in a relativist ontology and epistemology. Reality is not something that exists objectively and

independently of the stakeholders; reality is instead multiple and constructed. See also Thomas & Palfrey on stakeholder-focused evaluation (1996).

(3) *The concept of negotiated process and outcomes* As far as practicable, all the stakeholders (or their representatives) should be involved in all stages of the evaluation process. The process should be a collaborative one, not one imposed by managers or a single group of professionals.

(4) *The notion of evaluation as a continuous and divergent process* Evaluations are never fully completed. As some questions are answered, more questions emerge.

(5) *The notion of evaluation as an emergent process with unpredictable outcomes* Traditional evaluation approaches require that a design for an evaluation should be specified beforehand: in FGE the design, to some extent, unfolds as one progresses and as stakeholders' claims, concerns and issues are explored.

In this new evaluation world, evaluators need an array of capabilities over and above the traditional competences relating to validity and reliability in the collection and analysis of data. When undertaking FGE, evaluators need to appreciate diversity, to have a high tolerance for ambiguity and to have political skills of a high order. Guba & Lincoln (1989) do not see FGE as a competitor or replacement for earlier forms of evaluation; instead, they see it as subsuming them while moving to a higher level of sophistication and utility.

What are the practical implications of FGE for managers and health care professionals when setting out to evaluate a particular policy or service? They need to address the following questions:

- In deciding what to evaluate and how, have we taken sufficient account of the diverse perspectives and values of various stakeholders? For example, managers might see efficiency as the main issue, while health care professionals might focus more on effectiveness.

- Even with a single criterion there might be different emphases; for example, when judging effectiveness different stakeholders might have different objectives. So whose objectives 'count' when judging effectiveness?

- When managers and health care professionals set out to evaluate a service, to what extent will the views of others be taken into account in planning the evaluation? For example, patients and their relatives might have different perspectives about what is important in health care from those of managers.

- Have we recognised that evaluations are rarely 'complete'? Commonly, as some questions are answered so others are raised for further consideration. Within the resource constraints do we have an open mind on continuous improvement and evaluation?

- Are we paying enough attention to the concerns, claims and issues of all the key stakeholders?

The outpatient department in a general hospital is to be scrutinised by the managers as part of its internal quality audit. Managers are keen to ensure that members of the public are able to have access to an initial consultation within 40 minutes of registering at reception (output/ efficiency criteria).

While acknowledging that waiting times are important, members of the public stress the importance of being greeted courteously by the receptionist (process/acceptability criteria) and of being able to wait in a comfortable environment input/appropriateness criteria).

Clinical staff, on the other hand, are likely to place value on the adequacy of staffing, support and facilities in order to provide a 'good quality' service (input/acceptability criteria).

Laughlin & Broadbent (1996) are sceptical about Guba & Lincoln's ontological and epistemological position and are unhappy about what they see as their treatment of various stakeholders, giving, in their view, too much weight to the perspectives of clients and evaluators as opposed, say, to the perspectives of the staff delivering the services in question – perspectives which are given more weight by Caulley's 'fifth-generation' evaluation (1994).

Guba & Lincoln's argument that what is observed to be 'reality' is likely to tell us something about the observer as well as about the observed is not a particularly extreme view; it represents a position whose philosophical foundations are now well established (see, for example, Denzin & Lincoln, eds, 1994). Despite the criticisms, Guba & Lincoln's notion of fourth-generation evaluation represents a useful and important contribution to the evaluation literature.

Realistic evaluation

Another important contribution is that developed by Pawson & Tilley (1997). As Ho (1999) has pointed out, governmental evaluations have not always been sufficiently theory driven; that is, little understanding has been developed in relation to why and how programmes work. Pawson & Tilley's approach of 'realistic evaluations' addresses the questions of how, and in what circumstances, and for whom, does a programme work, and why, rather than simply collecting data to see whether a particular goal has been achieved. Their framework focuses on a programme's *context*, the programme's intervention *mechanism* and the particular *outcomes* for various stakeholders. This is an important framework because 'the operation of mechanisms is always contingent on context' (Pawson & Tilley, 1997, p. 216).

The argument is that experimental evaluations such as randomised controlled trials (the so called 'gold standard' of evaluation methods) cannot reveal enough about how and why particular interventions work. Experiments can usefully provide information about the extent to which an intervention such as a drug seems to give rise to particular outcomes, but they do not give sufficient guidance on the ways in which the interventions might be affected by variations in context, especially when 'policies' (rather than specific clinical interventions) are being evaluated. Experimental designs produce 'black box' evaluations (Bickman, 1987, in Clarke, 1999) in which change is measured by simply taking account of inputs and outputs while controlling for extraneous and intervening variables. But black box evaluations are thought to be 'unable to provide any real insight into the underlying causal mechanisms that produce treatment effects' (Clarke, 1999, p. 52). This should not normally be a problem when evaluating well defined and carefully controlled interventions such as drugs, but when we are evaluating more amorphous 'policies' Pawson & Tilley are right in calling for more 'theory driven' evaluations so that we can move towards a more comprehensive understanding of the *ways* in which policies are producing their apparent outcomes in particular situations.

Pawson & Tilley argue that more needs to be understood about the nature of causality in evaluations. They do accept that methods of data collection and analysis need to be 'appropriate' for the particular task; they are thus 'pluralistic' as far as research methods are concerned. But what concerns them is the need to delve beneath the surface to develop understandings of *why* and *how* policies work; evaluators 'need to penetrate beneath the surface of observable inputs and outputs of a program' (1997, p. 216).

Summary

In this chapter we have tried to show that evaluation is a crucial, indeed an inevitable and inherent, part of the work of health care professionals and managers. Parts of the chapter offer what we see as a useful model (summarised in Figure 1.1) for analysing important aspects of evaluation processes, while others offer prescriptive guidance on how evaluations 'should' be carried out. For example, managers and professionals need to be explicit about the criteria they are using when making judgements (evaluations) about how successfully, or otherwise, a policy, programme or service is working. We have also reviewed what seem to us to be some of the main issues relating to evaluation for health care professionals and managers. In the remainder of the book we examine a range of 'evaluative' issues which impinge on their work.

In Chapter 2, we examine the nature of 'management' within the health service before proceeding, in Chapter 3, to analyse the notion of 'multiple rationalities' which we see as a key issue in evaluation processes. In Chapter 4 we explore aspects of performance management within health care settings and some of the tools which are currently used in seeking to evaluate and improve the performance of health care agencies. In Chapter 5 our emphasis changes to some aspects of clinical and 'evidence-based' evaluations, and Chapter 6 analyses some of the political and ethical issues in health service evaluations. We then conclude, in Chapter 7, to offer some ideas about possible future directions for evaluation processes within the health service.

References

Ashburner, L. (2001) *Organisational Behaviour and Organisational Studies in Health Care: reflections on the future.* Palgrave, Basingstoke.

Audit Commission (2002) *Integrated Services for older people: Building a whole system approach in England.*

Bachrach, P. & Baratz, M. (1963) 'Decisions and nondecisions: an analytical framework'. *American Political Science Review*, **56** (57), 1947–52.

Baggott, R. (1998) *Health and Health Care in Britain.* Macmillan, London.

Bickman, L. (1987) *Using Program Theory in Evaluation.* Jossey-Bass, San Francisco.

Booth, T. (1981) 'Collaboration between the health and social services'. *Policy and Politics*, **9** (1), 23–49, and (2), 205–26.

Burrell, G. & Morgan, G. (1979) *Sociological Paradigms and Organisational Analysis.* Heinemann, London.

Caulley, D. (1994) 'Overview of Approaches to Program Evaluation: the Five generations' cited in Denzin & Lincoln (1994).

Challis, L., Fuller, S., Henwood, M., Klein, R., Plowden, W., Webb, A., Whittingham, P. & Wistow, G. (1988) *Joint Approaches to Social Policy.* Cambridge University Press, Cambridge.

Checkland, P. (1981) *Systems thinking, systems practice.* Wiley, London.

Clarke, A. (1999) *Evaluation Research: an introduction to principles, methods and practice.* Sage, London.

Davies, H. & Nutley, S. (2000) 'Healthcare: evidence to the fore', cited in Davies, Nutley & Smith (2002).

Davies, H., Nutley, S. & Smith, P. (2002) *What Works: Evidence-based policy and practice in public services.* Policy Press, Bristol.

Davies, P. (2000) 'Contributions from qualitative research', cited in Davies, Nutley & Smith (2002).

Denzin, N. & Lincoln, Y. (1994) *Handbook of Qualitative Research.* Sage, London.

Department of Health (1992) *The Health of the Nation: a strategy for Health in England* (Cm 1986) HMSO, London.

Easton, D. (1965) *A Systems Analysis of Political Life.* Wiley, New York.

Guba, E. & Lincoln, Y. (1989) *Fourth Generation Evaluation.* Sage, Newbury Park.

Hill, M. (1997) *The Policy Process in the Modern State.* Prentice, Hall & Wheatsheaf, London.

Ho, S.Y. (1999) 'Evaluating Urban Regeneration Programmes in Britain'. *Evaluation*, **5** (4), 422–38.

Hudson, B., Hardy, B., Henwood, M. & Wistow, G. (1999) 'In Pursuit of Inter-Agency Collaboration in the Public Sector'. *Public Management*, **1** (2), 235–60.

Huxham, C. (1996) *Creating Collaborative Advantage.* Sage, London.

Laughlin, R. & Broadbent, J. (1996) 'Redesigning Fourth-Generation Evaluation: an Evaluation Model for the Public Sector Reforms in the Public Sector'. *Evaluation*, **2** (4), 431–51.

Lindblom, C. (1959) 'The Science of "muddling through"'. *Public Administrative Review*, **19**, 78–88.

Lindblom, C. (1979) 'Still muddling, not yet through'. *Public Administrative Review*, **39**, 517–25.

Mark, A. (2001) Organising Emotional Health, cited in Ashburner (2001).

Maxwell, R. (1984) 'Quality assessment in health care'. *British Medical Journal*, **288**, 166–203.

National Assembly for Wales (2001) *Improving Health in Wales: a Plan for the NHS and its Partners.*

Palfrey, C., Phillips, C. & Thomas, P. (1991) *Efficiency, Economy and the Quality of Care.* Social Care Monograph, University of East Anglia.

Pawson, R. & Tilley, N. (1997) *Realistic Evaluation.* Sage, London.

Phillips, C. (2002) 'And all because the doctor prescribed an NSAID: Expenditure on PPIs and joined-up thinking in prescribing'. *British Journal of Health Care Management*, **8** (7), 272–5.

Phillips, C., Palfrey, C. & Thomas, P. (1994) *Evaluating Health and Social Care.* Macmillan, London.

Phillips, C. & Prowle, M. (1993) 'The economics of a reduction in smoking: A case study from Heartbeat Wales'. *Journal of Epidemiology and Community Health*, **47** (3), 215–23.

Rossi, P. & Freeman, H. (1993) *Evaluation: A Systematic Approach*. Sage, Newbury Park.

Senge, P. (1990) *The Fifth Discipline: the Art and Practice of the Learning Organisation*. Doubleday, New York.

Simon, H. (1957) *Administrative Behaviour*. Macmillan, New York.

Smith, G. & Cantley, C. (1985) *Assessing Health Care: a study in organisational evaluation*. Open University Press, Milton Keynes.

Thomas, P. (1988) 'Decision making and the management of change in the NHS'. *Health Services Management*, June, 29.

Thomas, P. & Palfrey, C. (1996) 'Evaluation: stakeholder-focused criteria'. *Social Policy and Administration*, **30** (2), 125–42.

Vince, R. (2001) 'Power and Emotion in Organisational Learning'. *Human Relations*, **54** (10), 1325–51.

Webb, A. (1991) 'Coordination: a problem in public sector management'. *Policy and Politics*, **19** (4), 229–41.

Wistow, G. (1982) 'Collaboration between Health and Local Authorities: Why is it Necessary?' *Journal of Social Policy and Administration*, **16** (1), 44–62.

Chapter 2
The Nature of Health Care Management

The policy context

At the risk of stating the obvious, 'management' is not a new idea in health care systems. One might be tempted to think that the idea started with the publication of the influential Griffiths Report (DHSS, 1983) when the notion of 'general management' was advocated and developed. But health services in the UK have been planned, implemented, organised and evaluated in the public sector since the inception of the National Health Service on 5 July 1948.

Major initiatives and reforms have been undertaken at various times since 1948 (for example, the 1962 Hospital Plan), but since the 1970s the number of new systems, reorganisations and reforms seems to have escalated. In 1974 there was a major restructuring in which the integrated task of planning and delivering local health services was given to area health authorities. Thus the previous tripartite system in which hospitals, general practitioners and community health services were managed by three separate administrative systems became more (though not wholly) integrated. In 1976 the 'NHS Planning System' was launched and in 1982 another reorganisation took place based on ideas taken from two reports published in 1979: the Report of the Royal Commission on the NHS and the Government's consultative document *Patients First* (DHSS, 1979). The problems that were to be addressed by these reforms included the existence of too many tiers in the structure, too many administrators, a failure to take quick decisions and wasted money (DHSS, 1979, para. 3).

In 1983 the Griffiths Report was published (DHSS, 1983). The working group, chaired by Roy Griffiths, then Deputy

Chairman and Managing Director of Sainsbury's supermarket chain, found that there were still significant weaknesses in the management of the NHS and that the service lacked a clearly defined general management function. Management in the NHS at this time was still largely based on a model of consensus management (DHSS, 1979). The working group argued:

> Absence of this general management support means that there is no driving force seeking and accepting direct and personal responsibility for developing management plans, securing their implementation and monitoring actual achievement.

> (DHSS, 1983, p. 12)

The report emphasised the importance of having general managers at all levels in the service who would provide the leadership and the management of change that was needed and argued that medical practitioners 'must accept the management responsibility which goes with clinical freedom' (DHSS, 1983, p. 18). The Government responded by requiring health authorities to appoint general managers throughout the service and these were put in place during the mid-1980s. However, in due course it became clear that 'applying business practices to an organisation like the NHS is difficult because of the political environment in which these practices are introduced' (Ham, 1992, p. 35).

Furthermore there was increasing recognition (Ham, 1992) during the 1980s of a widening gap between the funds made available to the NHS by the Government and the amount of money needed to satisfy the increasing demands on the service given the ageing population, the technological innovations being developed (enabling more to be done for people if adequate resources were available) and the increasing public expectations of what the NHS should be able to do.

The 'big idea' which was adopted by the Government at this time, in an attempt to improve the performance of the service, was that of the 'internal market' (Enthoven, 1985). The Department of Health white paper *Working for Patients* (Department of Health, 1989) proposed a new set of NHS reforms. The paper set out the new arrangements in which hospitals and community health units (both of which were in due course to become NHS trusts – the main 'providers' of front-line health services) would be required to compete with each other for contracts from health authorities (HAs) and GP fundholders, who would be the purchasers or 'commissioners' of services. The idea was that in order to win and retain contracts, and therefore retain patients and money from the HAs, there would be pressure on the trusts to reduce costs and improve the quality of services. In the context of Hirschman's conceptual framework (1971) the idea of increasing the use of market forces in this way represented a shift from the 'voice' end of Hirschman's spectrum (advocating the use of democracy and accountability as ways of improving services) to the 'exit' idea of making parts of the system compete with each other in terms of costs and quality to prevent 'customers' (purchasers) from exiting their relationship with the provider and going elsewhere.

As Baggott pointed out (1998), evaluation of this market solution was complicated by the existence of other policy initiatives:

> Particular problems arise when trying to evaluate the impact of policies which appear contradictory. The internal market was at odds with other policies, such as The Patient's Charter and the Health of the Nation strategies. These initiatives sought to impose central standards, while the market approach emphasised decentralisation and entrepreneurialism.
>
> (1998, p. 195)

In 1997, the new Labour Government declared that the internal market and the reliance on 'competition' as the basis for improving performance in the NHS would come to an end (Department of Health, 1997). In their place would come a return to partnership, integration and the development of new structures to replace the health authorities. Primary care groups (local health groups in Wales, where they share geographical boundaries with the 22 local authorities in Wales), later to become primary care trusts or local health boards, would be constituted to emphasise the increasingly important role of primary care in the planning of health care. However, the extent to which competitive forces will actually be removed from the service in the long term remains a moot point. Many argue that the development of league tables and continued use of performance indicators (not to mention the policy of creating 'foundation hospitals' in England) make it difficult to ignore the imperative of competitiveness.

What is 'health care management'?

This question is deceptive. At one level one might just say that health care management (HCM) concerns the activities of managers within the health service. However, there are a number of issues, largely in relation to professional autonomy, that make the notion of HCM more complex than it would otherwise be.

Let us begin by briefly examining the meaning of 'management'. In one sense we are all 'managers' because we are commonly expected to take responsibility for making decisions about scarce resources, even if the only resource one has is time. But the common understanding of management involves 'people looking beyond themselves and exercising formal authority over the activities and performance of other people' (Mullins, 2002, p. 166). A well known analysis of the elements of management is that provided by Fayol (1949):

(1) Planning
    Depending on the context, this might be referred to as decision making, policy making or strategy formulation. It entails examining possible futures and deciding what needs to be achieved and how.

(2) Organising
    This involves the provision and configuration of the resources (including people and their time) needed to implement the plan.

(3) Command
    This is now an unfashionable (and for many an unacceptable) concept because it implies 'telling' people

what to do. In many organisations (especially in health services, where there are many groups claiming professional status and a degree of autonomy) people now expect, at the very least, to be consulted about what is to be done. The concept of command has been largely replaced by the more consultative notion of 'leadership'. But managers are still expected to ensure that people do what is needed to implement the agreed plans. We leave to one side for the moment the issue of who has 'agreed' with the plan.

(4) Coordination
This is the process of unifying and integrating parts of the organisation and its resources so that as far as possible people are seeking to achieve goals that are consistent with each other.

(5) Control
This is the process of monitoring progress in implementing the plans and making judgements about what needs to be done to keep the organisation and its activities 'on track'.

This five-fold classification of the elements of management is in some respects similar to the model which we introduced in Chapter 1. In Figure 1.1 on page 4 the two boxes on the right-hand side of the diagram (deciding goals and objectives, and selecting suitable means of achieving those goals) are represented by 'planning' in Fayol's model. The 'implement' phase in our model encompasses stages (2) to (4) in Fayol's classification. Fayol's 'control' equates to the process of 'evaluation' and feeding back the results of the evaluation as an input to future decision making. Fayol's model sounds rather rational in an oversimplified sense. Our model seeks to correct this by giving greater emphasis to 'extra-rational' variables such as incrementalism and value judgements.

One of the other problems with Fayol's model is that it seems to be rather prescriptive. It sounds rather like a list of activities that managers 'ought' to be undertaking. When researchers have looked at what managers actually do in practice a less tidy, more iterative, picture emerges, one in which the activities of managers tend to be varied and disjointed (Mintzberg, 1973, 1990; Luthans, 1988; Stewart, 1999).

One of the particular problems of 'managing' in health care systems is the difference in approaches generally taken by managers and health care 'professionals' (for example medical practitioners, nurses and professionals allied to medicine). A common tension in public service organisations like a national health care system is the potential conflict between professional and managerial orientations. Professional groups are often characterised by autonomy, a claim to exclusive expertise, the possession of legally enforceable procedures and codes of ethics which regulate members' behaviour, control over entry and control over training. Such a professional group claims to be serving society at large and they commonly have high social status; and in the NHS they are normally trained to assess the needs of *individual* patients and to plan care accordingly.

Managers on the other hand are expected to take a wider view and to think about patients *collectively* and to plan services by making the most 'efficient' use of resources. They will be held accountable for this process by their managers and so on up the hierarchical structure. For managers there is often an emphasis on consistency and the procedures that bureaucracies need in order to function effectively. The functional differences between professionals and managers become complicated by the fact that one member of staff might be both a professional and a manager. This commonly occurs in the health care profession, for example, when a medical practitioner or a nurse takes on an increasing range of managerial responsibilities as their career progresses. This issue is further discussed in Chapter 6.

In the UK over the last 20 years, there is some evidence that an increasing degree of power has shifted from the medical profession (Harrison & Pollitt, 1994; Laffin, 1998; Harrison & Miller, 1999). For example, some inroads have been made into their professional/clinical autonomy and into their emphasis on the medical model of health care, which emphasises *individual* patients as opposed to a more *collective* orientation which managers are usually expected to adopt. But Harrison & Pollitt have argued that there are some significant limits to the extent to which the shift can continue. For example:

- continuing ability of professional groups to resist managerial control
- it would not be in managers' interests to extend their influence into certain areas
- the interests of managers themselves are likely to become fragmented
- Government realisation that giving power to managers will not give them (the Government) relief from the underlying pressures in the health care system (the need for rationing)

There is a good deal of evidence that relations remain tense between managers and clinicians within the NHS. Davies & Harrison (2003) have found a relatively high degree of discontentment among medical practitioners, partly because of their dissatisfaction with their relationships with managers. And in a survey of doctor-manager relationships in 197 NHS trusts Davies *et al.* (2003) found a higher degree of dissatisfaction among doctors than managers. For example, 37% of clinical directors felt positive about the relationships compared with 76% of chief executives. One of the main reasons for the dissatisfaction felt by the clinicians was the imbalance of power between doctors and managers and the quality of managerial staff.

According to the Office of Health Economics (Yuen, 2000) the numbers of professional staff in UK hospitals changed substantially during the 1990s. Between 1988 and 1999 the number of hospital nurses decreased by 13%, the number of hospital doctors increased by 40%, and the number of general and senior managers in hospitals increased by 479%! Of course crude numbers of this sort can be misleading and can sometimes be partly accounted for by changing categories and definitions, but the figures suggest a growing emphasis on managerial processes within hospital services in the UK in recent years.

The 'balance of power' between the two groups (health care professionals/clinicians and health care managers) is a changing one (not necessarily always in the same direction) and will vary according to a wide range of contextual variables. It is likely to remain a fruitful area for empirical research in the foreseeable future.

Public versus private sector management

There are other issues which differentiate health care management and public sector management generally from generic management practice as it is commonly understood within private sector organisations of all kinds. Willcocks & Harrow (1992) have identified the following features of 'public management' generally:

- a greater degree of political accountability
- objectives and priorities that are often vague and/or conflicting
- complex networks of stakeholders
- less competition (though competitive forces are now not unknown in the NHS)
- the inevitability of rationing (insufficient resources to meet all demands)
- the professional autonomy of various employee groups
- a distinctive legal context

These issues make the task of health care managers in the public sector more complex than those faced by, perhaps, industrial and commercial managers. It also means that the task of evaluating performance becomes more difficult than it would otherwise be. In practice the evaluation process would require managers and professionals to address questions such as:

- whose objectives are to be given greatest weight?
- what degree of governmental involvement in the planning, implementation and evaluation of health policies is acceptable and appropriate?

- given that resources are never likely to be sufficient to meet all expectations, how explicit should health care staff be about the nature and degree of rationing?
- what should be the balance between managers' 'right to manage' and the need for health care professionals to retain an appropriate degree of clinical autonomy?

The skills, attributes and competences of managers

An early contribution to the literature on managerial skills was the work of Katz (1974), who argued that managers require a combination of technical competence, social and human skills and conceptual ability, with the last mentioned becoming increasingly important as managers reach more senior positions. A later and more detailed analysis was undertaken by Pedler *et al.* (1994), whose research indicated that successful managers possess eleven qualities grouped into three areas as follows:

Basic knowledge and information
- command of basic facts
- relevant professional understanding

Skills and attributes
- continuing sensitivity to events
- analytical, problem-solving, decision/judgement making skills
- social skills and abilities
- emotional resilience
- proactivity – indication to respond purposefully to events

'Meta-qualities'
- creativity
- mental agility
- balanced learning habits and skills
- self-knowledge

Pedler and his colleagues provide a useful diagnostic exercise which can help managers to diagnose their strengths and development needs in relation to these eleven qualities. The framework has been used for many years as a part of management development programmes for health care managers.

More recently, Hamlin (2002) has used critical incident technique and factor analysis methods to identify a range of positive and negative criteria of competent managers in a case study of an NHS trust hospital. The managers studied were 'middle managers' and 'first time' managers. Furthermore, Hamlin has undertaken a comparison with studies in other public sector organisations and argues that the lists of identified criteria have generalised universal relevance distinct from a contingency approach in which such universalism is rejected in favour of more situation-specific analyses. The lists are as follows (Hamlin, 2002, p. 255):

Positive criteria
- organisation and planning
- active supportive leadership
- giving support to staff
- open and personal management approach or style
- inclusive decision making
- looking after the interests and needs of staff
- empowerment and delegation
- informing people

Negative criteria
- dictatorial/autocratic management
- intimidating staff
- negative approach
- undermining of others
- avoidance and ignoring behaviour
- failing to inform other people
- not giving, receiving or using information
- exhibiting poor organisation
- self serving and uncaring management
- lack of concern for staff
- abdicating roles and responsibilities

An even more detailed analysis of what managers are thought to do is that used in the 'competence' movement. In 1988 the Management Charter Initiative was launched. Set up by employers with the support of the Government, the

MCI has pioneered the competence approach to developing and assessing what managers should be able to do, by introducing national 'management standards' which can be used as 'benchmarks of best practice used by managers' (Mullins, 2002, p. 857). The standards currently comprise seven key 'roles' which relate to the management of:

- activities
- resources
- people
- information
- energy
- quality
- projects

Each of these seven roles is subdivided in turn into 'units', and each unit into 'elements'. The detail of what managers are expected to be able to do in relation to each element is then made explicit in a range of 'performance criteria', and is underpinned with a range of specific 'knowledge and understanding' that managers are expected to be able to demonstrate.

However, the competence approach and the use of management standards are not without their critics. In particular, reducing management to a set of highly specific 'elements' and performance criteria is thought by some to be too mechanistic and reductionist in its approach (Jones & Thomas, 1994, pp. 8–12). Rather, it has been argued that management needs to be seen holistically as a more complex and synergistic process. Nevertheless, management development programmes for health care managers have been shown to work 'successfully' in the views of the trainees themselves, using the competence approach, especially when used in combination with more conventionally academic approaches which require more conceptual and reflective work – a 'mixed model' of management development (Jones & Thomas, 1994; Williams *et al.*, 2000, pp. 571–4).

The professional institute for health care managers in the UK (the Institute of Healthcare Management) has published a management code which sets out the Institute's approach to education and development of health care managers. It includes the MCI standards as one of the approaches available to managers and emphasises that 'continuing professional development' is now mandatory for IHM members. The management code also stresses the importance of the principles elaborated by the Committee on Standards in Public Life (Nolan Committee, 1995; see also Chapter 6): selflessness, integrity, objectivity, accountability, openness, honesty and leadership. For each of the principles the code sets out the behaviour patterns of an 'excellent manager' and of an 'unacceptable manager'. For example, in relation to *accountability* the 'excellent manager':

- acts after careful consideration of the consequences in the best interests of patients and the organisation
- complies with statutory requirements but utilises discretion
- consults widely before taking action with major impact

The 'unacceptable manager' on the other hand:

- acts by reflex without considering the consequences
- is very superficial in approach to planning
- dismisses the effect on others

What are the implications of this for health care managers? The relatively recent development of approaches which explicitly specify particular 'behaviour patterns' and/or competences means that managers have a choice when planning or supporting management development programmes. Should managers be assessed in relation to portfolios of evidence of specific competences in their day-to-day managerial life or should more traditional academic approaches be used (for example, essays, examinations and projects/dissertations)? The choice will influence the kind of management training and development to be used.

The way forward is likely to involve striking a balance between the two approaches. It does not need to be a straight choice between a university course leading to a postgraduate degree on the one hand or an NVQ 4 or 5 in management on the other. Judicious and flexible choices will need to be made at various times according to the career trajectory of the manager concerned and the changing priorities of the service. This requires a careful needs analysis (the box at the top of Figure 1.1 in Chapter 1 on page 4). The competence approach to analysing managerial activities is also commonly thought to contrast sharply with the more holistic model of 'reflective practice' to which we now turn.

Health care managers as reflective practitioners

In Chapter 1 we summarised some of the main features of Guba & Lincoln's notion of fourth-generation evaluation. One of their concerns is to promote a relativist ontology and epistemology. They argue that reality is not something that exists objectively and independently of stakeholders: reality is instead multiple and constructed. This view has received much support in recent years by researchers who acknowledge the value and usefulness of positivism but who also see its limitations (for example, see Chia, 1997; Ashburner 2001; Kember *et al.*, 2001). The debate is commonly traced back to Schon's promotion of the idea of 'reflective practice' (1983, 1987). Schon challenges what he sees as the inappropriately dominant epistemology (positivism and technical rationality) and argues for an approach which encourages professionals to reflect on their practice and learning as they carry out their work. As we argue elsewhere in this book, especially in Chapters 3 and 5, professionals also need to remain sensitive to the views, values and preferences of the various stakeholders involved in any decision arena.

One of the reasons that Schon gives for the change in orientation is that problems faced by professionals exist at two levels: the high ground and the low ground. For the last couple of centuries a hegemony of positivism and technical rationality has dominated the world of research on the professions (science, technology, medicine, etc.). It is on this 'high ground' that the problems of society are well defined. However, many of the problems which need to be examined through reflective practice and action research are in what Schon (1987, p. 3) calls the 'swampy lowlands'. In the swampy lowlands, problems are messy and confusing and they defy technical solutions. The problem is that many of our most important problems are in the swamp.

> The problems of real world practice do not present them-selves to practitioners as well-formed structures. Indeed they tend not to present themselves as problems at all but as messy, indeterminate situations. Civil engineers, for example, know how to build roads suited to the conditions of particular sites and specifications. They draw on their knowledge of soil conditions, materials, and construction technologies to define grades, surfaces and dimensions. When they must decide what road to build, however, or whether to build at all, their problem is not solvable by the application of technical knowledge, not even by the sophisticated techniques of decision theory. They face a complex and ill-defined melange of topographical, financial, economic, environmental and political factors.
>
> (Schon, 1987, p. 4)

The idea of reflective practice (and the related approach of action research) to deal with 'messy' problems has been influential in a number of health care professions. Kember and his colleagues (2001) have used the approach in the education and training of a range of health care professionals (post experience nurses, clinical educators, physiotherapists, occupational therapists and radiographers). Their aim was 'to enable students in the health professions to fully combine the theory aspect of their courses with the professional practice element by encouraging them to adopt reflective practice' (2001, p. vii). Hart & Bond (1995) have also demonstrated the value of reflective and action research approaches in a wide range of health care settings (including management), as have Winter & Munn-Giddings (2001).

It is difficult, and probably inappropriate, to try to offer a simple prescription about how professionals and managers should utilise reflective practice (RP) as a means of develop-ing their expertise and capabilities. The book by Kember *et al.* (2001) is a good starting point for people who want to see how the approach has been used in the education and training of a wide range of health care professionals. Among their ideas for operationalising RP are the following elements:

- the need to reflect critically on what one does as a practitioner (as a manager or health care professional) and on what happens as a result of one's practice
- a regular re-examination of one's experience, beliefs and conceptual knowledge
- the generation of new perspectives and knowledge arising from reflections *on* action (reflecting *after* one's actions) and reflection *in* action (reflecting *during* one's actions)
- the welcoming of challenges to one's standard way of thinking about and acting on problems

Many of the problems with which managers and professionals in health care systems have to deal are 'messy' but this does not mean that we are arguing that positivism has had its day. And we are certainly not arguing that other paradigms are 'better' for understanding, researching and practising management, evaluation and other 'messy' work in health care settings. But we welcome the development of alternative 'interpretive' approaches which can sometimes be used to complement the more traditional positivist paradigm and which for many problems are likely to be the more appropriate way forward (Burrell & Morgan, 1979).

This does not mean that managers cannot base their management practice on 'evidence'. After all, as Walshe & Rundall point out (2001), if medical practitioners are expected by managers to pursue evidence-based clinical practice, the clinicians could be forgiven for expecting managers to pursue evidence-based practice in health care management, an issue to which we turn in Chapter 3. However, there are a number of problems in getting managers to adopt this kind of approach (Walshe & Rundall, 2001). To begin with there are striking cultural differences between the worlds occupied by clinicians and managers. Clinicians are, because of their training and career development paths, generally far more at home with dealing with research projects and their results than are most managers, who form a more heterogeneous group. Second, the evidence available to clinicians tends to be based on a strong biomedical, empirical paradigm where results are normally expected to have general applicability. Managers on the other hand have more difficulty finding easily applicable generalisable research, partly because in managerial and organisational matters, contextual and confounding variables are more complicated. Third, many clinical decisions are taken by individual clinicians, whereas managers are more likely to find they have far less autonomy, sandwiched as they often are between organisational and political pressures (the 'incremental' box in the middle of Figure 1.1 on page 4 in Chapter 1).

Walshe & Rundall (2001) go on to describe an initiative in the USA which seeks to help managers to access, understand and utilise an increasing 'evidence base' related to health care management problems. The idea of 'evidence-based management' is being further developed by the Center for Health Management Research (CHMR) which was founded in 1992 by a consortium of health care organisations and academic centres (Thomas Rundall at the University of California is co-director of CHMR). The goals of CHMR are:

- to develop a research agenda in collaboration with corporate members
- to undertake research, development and evaluation projects on behalf of the corporate members
- to disseminate to the members the findings of health services research
- to identify and disseminate to the members successful innovations and management practices from other health care organisations
- to identify and disseminate to the members relevant research findings of successful innovations and management practices from other industries

(Walshe & Rundall, 2001, pp. 446–7)

The need is for the results of high quality management research to be summarised and disseminated to managers in easy-to-use formats and in journals they are likely to read.

This is an interesting and potentially useful development but as they point out 'this kind of cultural and attitudinal change is unlikely to happen quickly' (Walshe & Rundall, 2001, p. 452). Nevertheless, in the long term it is 'surely in the interests of all stakeholders in the health care system to have better, more evidence-based processes for making managerial decisions and developing health care policy' (Walshe & Rundall, 2001, p. 453). We return to the issue of evidence-based practice in Chapter 5.

Future directions for health care management

Governments continue to introduce reforms and structural reorganisations in an apparently never-ending series of changes to the ways in which the NHS is managed. Although the Labour Government declared that there was to be a shift away from the internal market and a move back towards collaboration and partnerships (Department of Health, 1997; Welsh Office, 1998) it is not entirely clear that the days of 'competition' are over in the NHS. As we have noted earlier, the emergence of foundation hospitals is seen by some as a potentially divisive mechanism which is likely to lead to a two-tier system, with hospitals keen to gain foundation status in order to attain greater autonomy and attract greater numbers of patients, and therefore money. This, together with the increasing use of league tables, performance indicators and star ratings, is seen by some as evidence that 'competitive forces are still seen by government as a useful means of driving up performance' (Carvel, 2003).

In its blueprint for the new foundation hospitals (Department of Health, 2002a) the Government make it clear that they see these new hospitals as staying clearly within the NHS and as staying faithful to the underlying values of the service. But it does seem that a more varied and pluralistic model of public health care is emerging. The then Secretary of State for Health (Alan Milburn) in announcing his plans for a reformed NHS believed that it did not matter that some patients might be treated in a BUPA hospital or a foundation hospital. The patients will remain NHS patients because 'the NHS is not its bricks and mortar. It is fundamentally a set of values' (*The Times*, 20 April 2002). At the same time the main commissioning bodies in recent years (health authorities) have been replaced by primary care groups/trusts (Department of Health, 2002b) who, in England, will have annual performance agreements with new 'strategic health authorities'.

In 2002 the Government also published new guidance to NHS managers about their role in the changing health service (Department of Health, 2002c). In *Managing for Excellence in the NHS* the Department of Health set out the three components of the 'new management task' (2002c, p. 5) on which managers were increasingly expected to focus:

- partnerships in managing clinical processes and service delivery, a recognition that clinicians and health service managers do not always see eye to eye on how services should be planned and delivered
- full engagement with patients, staff and local communities, including an outward accountability through mechanisms such as patients' forums
- new skills to deliver lasting change

As far as the last of these points is concerned, the paper spells out the 'core skills' which are required (Department of Health, 2002c, p. 8):

- managing people
- managing information
- managing resources
- managing communications

This classification is similar to that used by the MCI in relation to managerial competences referred to earlier in this chapter. But the paper also suggests that in future there needs to be a greater focus on such management processes as:

- engaging with patients, clinicians and local communities at all levels
- changing behaviours
- working with local stakeholders and politicians
- measured risk taking
- contributing to and leading partnerships
- working across organisational boundaries

The last two of these issues clearly point to the need for health service managers and others to become more effective at what is sometimes called 'joined-up' thinking. The problem of getting organisations to collaborate with each other effectively in order to achieve a seamless or joined-up delivery of services is a long-standing one (see, for example, Wistow, 1982; Benson, 1983; Challis *et al.*, 1988; Wistow & Brooks, 1988; Palfrey *et al.*, 1991; Webb, 1991; Bryson & Crosby, 1992; Huxham, 1996; Huxham, 2000; El Ansari *et al.*, 2001).

In this context, Goodwin & Shapiro (2002) have recently re-emphasised the obstacles to integrated primary care and social services, such as conflicting priorities between the agencies concerned. They argue for the need to develop a greater degree of sharing of issues, funding, planning and service delivery. Hudson *et al.* (1999) have argued that inter-agency collaboration in the public sector remains chronically difficult, yet governments understandably remain enthusiastic about it: 'indeed, if anything, the pursuit of inter-agency collaboration has become hotter' (1999, p. 236). Hudson and his colleagues have developed a conceptual framework setting out what they see as the main issues that need to be considered when planning collaborative services. The framework contains the following elements (see also Jones *et al.*, 2004):

(1) contextual factors: expectations and constraints
    This group of factors recognises that problems can rarely be solved by organisations working individually. In order to reduce the incidence of unnecessary duplication and conflict, organisations are increasingly expected to work together. Thus organisations might be able to achieve 'collaborative advantage' if the acknowledged limits of organisational individualism and the virtues of collaboration are recognised.

(2) Recognition of the need to collaborate
    An issue closely related to the first is that the need for collaboration is reinforced in order to reduce the more dysfunctional symptoms of conflict. However, there are also potential drawbacks to collaborative activity. They

include the need to invest resources in developing collaborative relationships and the possibility of losing (or sharing) any individual credit that might be available for work well done jointly. As Hudson *et al.* point out, 'collaborative initiatives will not arise easily nor be self-perpetuating' (1999, p. 242).

(3) Identification of a legitimate basis for collaboration
Exchange theory assumes that self-interest underpins most organisational activity (Blau, 1964). The resource dependency model (Benson, 1983) focuses on the need for people and organisations to see that it can be in their interests to persevere with collaborative activity. The more likely it is that people can see a potential net benefit for themselves in engaging in collaboration, the more likely it is for them to do so.

(4) Assessment of collaborative capacity
The development of an appropriate culture is a prerequisite for effective collaboration. One of the difficulties is that while prescriptive collaborative documents commonly begin by stating a set of unifying values the reality is often the existence of conflicting values. 'Culture is something that the organisation *is* rather than a variable that can be manipulated by management' (Hudson, 1999, p. 246). A careful assessment is needed of organisations' collaborative capacity.

(5) Articulation of a clear sense of collaborative purpose
It can too easily be taken for granted that an explicit statement of shared vision is a prerequisite to collaborative success. But several scholars have pointed out that *too* explicit a statement can be unhelpful. Pettigrew *et al.* (1992), for example, have argued that for a starting point a broad vision may be more likely to generate movement than a blueprint. In the world of politics and negotiation, ambiguity is commonly a useful facilitator.

(6) Building up trust from principled conduct
The aim should be 'collaborative sustainability' (Cropper, 1995), a kind of virtuous circle in which a

level of *sufficient* trust enables a start to be made which may lead to a sufficiently successful outcome to reinforce future collaborative commitment.

(7) Ensuring wide organisational ownership
This entails recognising and nurturing 'reticulists' (those who are skilled at developing and exploiting networks), and securing the commitment of front line staff – Lipsky's 'street level bureaucrats' (1980).

(8) Nurturing fragile relationships
It is important to recognise that because of, for example, resistance to change, collaborative activity can be fragile and vulnerable to the actions and omissions of vested interests. In practice one probably needs to proceed incrementally, but preferably with a longer term goal in mind. This is akin to Bryson's notion of 'thinking big and acting small' (Bryson, 1988).

(9) Selection of an appropriate collaborative relationship
There are various kinds and degrees of collaborative relationships. There is no 'one right way' and one needs to develop a relationship with partners which is appropriate to the particular context, for example, in relation to the patterns of accountability to the various partner organisations, which are expected.

(10) Selection of a coordination pathway
Again there are choices. Is what is required a market framework, more hierarchical arrangements or a network system?

We believe that this model provides a useful device for analysing the need for, and feasibility of, achieving joined-up services, but as Hudson *et al.* point out, there need to be empirical studies in order to test the model's robustness. This can be done in any forum where managers and professionals need to work across organisational boundaries to achieve positive health care outcomes, for example, the planning and implementation of hospital discharge policies or the care for the mentally ill. The task of achieving effective joined-up

planning and delivery of health services (through partnerships, networks, joint committees or other devices) is likely
to remain one of the key challenges in health care for the
foreseeable future.

Summary

What does all this mean for the health care manager? To
begin with there is a need to fully recognise the unique features of public sector management to which we have drawn
attention in this chapter. Where managers are appointed
from outside the public service it can come as quite a shock
to them to discover the extent to which the health service is
politically charged. 'Simple' apolitical management models
are less likely to work than they are in the private sector. This
is further complicated in the health service by the implicit,
and sometimes explicit, competition between 'managers' and
'professionals' for influence over the planning, implementation
and evaluation of services.

Related to this is the need for health care managers to
monitor their own development in terms of what they are
expected to be capable of. Continuing professional development (CPD) frameworks can help managers to seek and
achieve continuous performance improvement in the NHS
but the road is likely to remain a bumpy and uncertain one.
Increasing expectations that management will become more
evidence-based will be difficult to meet, especially given the
complex nature of managerial and policy issues within the
NHS.

Of particular importance is the need to find innovative
ways of achieving and maintaining partnerships and collaborative ways of working so that the various agencies whose
work impinges on health can work together in more appropriate and effective ways. This has been a long-standing problem but the need for solving it remains a critical task. The
problem includes the tensions that persist between national
policy initiatives such as national service frameworks and
guidance from NICE in order to reduce the phenomenon of

'postcode prescribing' on the one hand and expectations that health services should respond to locally determined needs on the other.

Finally, given that the pace of reform and change continues to dominate managerial agendas, the need for managers to develop their ability to plan, implement and evaluate change has never been greater. The inevitable pluralistic nature of the management task in the NHS, in which differences of opinion about how services should be planned, implemented and evaluated are inevitable, serves to emphasise the importance of the 'incrementalist' and 'value judgement' elements of our model (see Figure 1.1, on page 4, Chapter 1). It is to the pluralistic nature of health care management and its multiple rationalities that we now turn.

References

Ashburner, L. (2001) *Organisational Behaviour and Organisational Studies in Health Care: reflections on the future*. Palgrave, Basingstoke.

Baggott, R. (1998) *Health and Health Care*. Macmillan, London.

Benson, J. (1983) 'Inter-organisational networks and Policy Sectors', cited in Rogers & Whetter (1983).

Blau, P. (1964) *Exchange and Power in Social Life*. John Wiley, New York.

Bryson, J. (1988) 'Strategic Planning: Big Wins and Small Wins'. *Public Money and Management*, Autumn, 11–15.

Bryson, J. & Crosby, B. (1992) *Leadership for the Common Good: Tackling Public Problems in a Shared-Power World*. Jossey Bass, San Francisco.

Burrell, G. & Morgan, G. (1979) *Sociological Paradigms and Organisational Analysis*. Heinemann, London.

Carvel, J. (2003) 'NHS hospitals forced to compete for patients'. *Guardian*, 6 March 2003.

Challis, L., Fuller, S., Henwood, M., Klein, R., Plowden, W., Webb, A., Whittingham, P. & Wistow, G. (1988) *Joint Approaches to Social Policy*. Cambridge University Press, Cambridge.

Chia, R. (1997) 'Essai: Thirty Years On: From Organisational Structures to the Organisation of Thought'. *Organisation Studies*, **18** (4), 685–707.

Cropper, S. (1995) 'Collaborative Working and the Issue of Sustainability', cited in Huxham (1996).

Davies, H. & Harrison, S. (2003) 'Trends in doctor-manager relationships'. *British Medical Journal*, **326**, 646–9.

Davies, H., Hodges, C. & Rundall, T. (2003) 'Views of doctors and managers on the doctor-manager relationship in the NHS'. *British Medical Journal*, **326**, 626–8.

Department of Health (1989) *Working for Patients*. (Cm 555) HMSO, London.

Department of Health (1997) *The new NHS: Modern, Dependable*. (Cm 3807) HMSO, London.

Department of Health (2002a) *Guide to NHS Foundation Trusts*. HMSO, London.

Department of Health (2002b) *Shifting the Balance of Power: the next steps*. HMSO, London.

Department of Health (2002c) *Managing for Excellence in the NHS*. HMSO, London.

Department of Health and Social Security (1979) *Patients First*. HMSO, London.

Department of Health and Social Security (1983) *NHS Management Inquiry*. (The Griffiths Report), Department of Health and Social Security, London.

El Ansari, W., Phillips, C. & Hammick, M. (2001) 'Collaboration and partnerships: developing the evidence base'. *Health and Social Care in the Community*, **9** (4), 215–27.

Enthoven, A. (1985) *Reflections on the management of the NHS*. Nuffield Provincial Hospital Trusts, London.

Fayol, H. (1949) *General and Industrial Management*. Pitman, London.

Goodwin, N. & Shapiro, J. (2002) 'The Road to Success'. *Health Management*, March, 20–22.

Guba, E. & Lincoln, Y. (1989) *Fourth-Generation Evaluation*. Sage, Newbury Park.

Ham, C. (1992) *Health Policy in Britain: the politics and organisation of the National Health Service*. Macmillan, London.

Hamlin, R. (2002) 'A study and comparative analysis of managerial and leadership effectiveness in the National Health Service: an empirical factor analytical study within an NHS Trust hospital'. *Health Services Management Research*, **15**, 245–63.

Harrison, R. & Miller, S. (1999) 'The Contribution of Clinical Directors to the Strategic Capability of the Organisation'. *British Journal of Management*, **10**, 23–39.

Harrison, S. & Pollitt, C. (1994) *Controlling Health Professionals*. Open University Press, Milton Keynes.

Hart, E. & Bond, M. (1995) *Action research for health and social care: a guide to practice*. Open University Press, Milton Keynes.

Hirschman, A. (1971) *Exit, Voice and Loyalty: Responses to Decline of Firms, Organisations and States*. Harvard University Press, Massachusetts.

Hudson, B., Hardy, B., Henwood, M. & Wistow, G. (1999) 'In Pursuit of Inter-Agency Collaboration in the Public Sector'. *Public Management*, **1** (2), 235–60.

Huxham, C. ed. (1996) *Creating Collaborative Advantage*. Sage, London.

Huxham, C. (2000) 'The Challenge of Collaborative Governance'. *Public Management*, **2** (3), 337–57.

Jones, N. & Thomas, P. (1994) 'The MCI Approach to Crediting Competence: Towards a Mixed Model of Management Development'. *Training Matters*, **2**, 8–12.

Jones, N., Thomas, P. & Rudd, L. (2004) 'Collaborating for Mental Health Services in Wales: a process evaluation'. *Public Administration*.

Katz, R. (1974) 'Skills of an Effective Administrator'. *Harvard Business Review*, September–October, 90–102.

Kember, D., Jones, A., Yuen Loke, A. *et al.* (2001) *Reflective Teaching and Learning in the Health Professions*. Blackwell, London.

Laffin, M. ed. (1998) *Beyond Bureaucracy? The Professions in the Contemporary Public Sector*. Ashgate, Aldershot.

Lipsky, M. (1980) *Street Level Bureaucracy*. Russell Sage, New York.

Luthans, F. (1988) 'Successful versus Effective Real Managers'. *The Academy of Management Executive*, **11** (2), 127–32.

Mintzberg, H. (1973) *The Nature of Managerial Work*. Harper and Row, New York.

Mintzberg, H. (1990) 'The Manager's Job: Folklore and Fact'. *Harvard Business Review Classic*, March–April, 163–76.

Mullins, L. (2002) *Management and Organisational Behaviour*. Pearson, Harlow.

Nolan Committee (1995) Standards in Public Life. HMSO, London.

Palfrey, C., Phillips, C. & Thomas, P. (1991) *Efficiency, Economy and the Quality of Care*. Social Care Monograph, University of East Anglia.

Pedler, M., Burgoyne, J. & Boydell, T. (1994) *A Manager's Guide to Self-Development*. McGraw-Hill, London.

Pettigrew, A., Ferlie, E. & McKee, L. (1992) *Shaping Strategic Change*. Sage, London.

Rogers, D. & Whetter, D. (1983) *Interorganisational Coordination*. Iowa State University Press, Iowa.

Royal Commission on the National Health Service (1979) Cmnd. 7615. HMSO (the Merrison Report), London.

Schon, D. (1983) *The Reflective Practitioner: how Professionals Think in Action*. Basic Books, New York.

Schon, D. (1987) *Educating the Reflective Practitioner: Towards a New Design for Teaching and Learning in the Professions*. Jossey-Bass, San Francisco.

Stewart, R. (1999) *The Reality of Management*. Butterworth Heinemann, London.

Walshe, K. & Rundall, T. (2001) 'Evidence-based management: From Theory to Practice in Health Care'. *The Milbank Quarterly*, **79** (3), 429–57.

Webb, A. (1991) 'Coordination: a problem in public sector management'. *Policy and Politics*, **19** (4), 229–41.

Welsh Office (1998) *NHS Wales: Putting Patients First*. Cmnd. 3841. HMSO, London.

Willcocks, L. & Harrow, J. (1992) *Rediscovering Public Management*. McGraw-Hill, London.

Williams, S., Thomas, P. & Emmerson, M. (2000) 'Reviewing the outcomes of "mixed model" development'. *British Journal of Health Care Management*, **6**, 12.

Winter, R. & Munn-Giddings, C. (2001) *A Handbook for Action Research in health and Social Care*. Routledge, London.

Wistow, G. (1982) 'Collaboration Between Health and Local Authorities: Why is it Necessary?' *Journal of Social Policy and Administration*, **16** (1), 44–62.

Wistow, G. & Brooks, T. (1988) *Joint Planning and Joint Management*. Royal Institute of Public Administration, London.

Yuen, P. (2000) *Compendium of Health Statistics*. Office of Health Economics, London.

Chapter 3
Multiple Perspectives and Decision Making

Introduction

Management decisions within the health care system have primarily to do with issues relating to resources and resource allocation. Managing budgets and managing people are two key managerial functions. Yet, as we have noted in the previous chapter, the UK Governments over the past three decades have considered it necessary to restructure the NHS in order to improve the quality of decision making.

Ever since its inception, accusations of inefficiency have been levelled at the health service. The introduction of prescription charges in the 1960s was an early indication that taxation and National Insurance levies alone would not sustain an expanding health care system. In effect, the Government of the day was conceding that its own management of the NHS was not proving entirely effective. This admission, though implicit rather than a public statement, serves to highlight an important consideration in any discussion of effective management in the health service – the potential tension between different levels of management.

In this chapter we concentrate on effective management at Government, strategic health authority, trust and primary care levels. Yet effective management can relate to central government decisions about the financing, structure and staff recruitment and retention within the NHS. Furthermore, Government criteria for evaluating the performance of different tiers within the health service can be imposed from above. Chapter 4 deals in some detail with a variety of indicators that have been and which are being applied in order to assess the quality of service provision. These are largely output indicators which involve a comparative approach in order to make judgements about performance: comparison over time, across different geographical regions and between similar organisations.

Managers within the NHS have, therefore, to serve a number of constituencies, which are likely to evaluate 'success' according to different yardsticks. For example, primary care trusts and local health boards will be answerable not only to Parliament or, in Wales, to the National Assembly, but to the communities which they are intended to serve. It will be interesting to observe how these bodies will function, with the potential to be both commissioners of health care services and providers. Executive members of these organisations also represent a range of vested interests – GPs, dentists, dieticians, optometrists as well as lay representatives from voluntary organisations.

Chief executives/directors will need to exhibit a range of competences and skills in order to reconcile and integrate differing perspectives on priority spending areas in both the budgetary and geographical senses of the word. Not least, they and the chairpersons will be held accountable and can be summarily dismissed by, respectively, the Director of the NHS in the four regions of the UK and by the Secretary of State or Minister for Health. Managers are going to be increasingly subject to competing rationalities, not least in attempting to reconcile the requirements to meet local health needs as well as meeting NSF targets and conforming to evidence-based directives from NICE.

Making rational decisions

An interesting debate in the USA in the 1950s centred on models of the policy making process. Simon (1957) depicted what was originally termed 'comprehensive rationality' as the method by which policies are and ought to be made. His preoccupation with a linear structure of decision making in his promotion of a process of policy making that followed sequentially logical stages was challenged by Lindblom (1959).

The incremental model, offered by Lindblom, disputed Simon's model and claimed that in the real world, policies were not created and implemented in a way that followed a step by step progression from defining the issue or problem; generating various options in order to deal with the issues; selecting the 'best' option and then implementing the eventual policy. Lindblom's contention was that policy making was more of a process of 'muddling through' in which key players tested out policy incrementally in a series of decisions resting on 'partisan mutual adjustment'. Decisions were tentative and subject to amendments in the light of experience.

In response to this alternative explanation of decision making at various levels Simon conceded that the 'best' option was not always available and that a next best alternative might need to be agreed. His prescriptive model appeared to be an 'ideal' type that was rarely achievable in the sphere of policy making As a compromise, Simon adjusted his earlier idea and reconstructed his model as one in which policy makers were confined by matters often outside their control. His model re-emerged as one of 'bounded rationality'.

According to this model, while 'economic man' maximises, or selects the best alternative from among all those available, 'administrative man' 'satisfices', or looks for a course of action that is 'good enough'. Objective rationality is bounded by three limitations:

- rationality requires a complete knowledge and anticipation of the consequences that will follow on each choice but knowledge of consequences is always fragmentary
- since these consequences lie in the future, imagination must supply the lack of experienced feeling in attaching value to them but values can only be imperfectly anticipated
- rationality requires a choice among all possible alternative behaviours but in actual behaviour, only a very few of all these possible alternatives ever come to mind

(Simon, 1957)

This attempt, and later efforts by Vickers (1965), Etzioni (1967), Challis *et al.* (1988) and Dror (1989), to present explanations and models of the policy making process, although interesting in the field of academic enquiry, might appear somewhat detached from the world of health care management. Their ideas do, however, bring into focus, at the very least, the question of what constitutes 'the best option' or 'second best option' in health care management decision making. In addition, attempts to construct both descriptive and prescriptive models of the policy making process direct our attention to the inevitably contextual relativity in which such models or ideal types have their origin.

During the mid-1980s, when Margaret Thatcher's Government was actively seeking ways to reform if not dismantle the NHS, the Prime Minister called upon a succession of advisers outside her Cabinet and Civil Service to help point the way to a more competitive, more efficient health service. One of these advisers was an American health economist Alain Enthoven. He advised Mrs Thatcher, later Lady Thatcher, to try out the proposed changes in one area of the UK. In so doing, he believed that any 'wrinkles' could be ironed out and changes made before the policy was implemented across the UK.

His reasoning was that the 'Big Bang' approach to policy making would not work because it was not the way it was done in the USA. However, despite a number of amendments to the original proposal to move towards a USA style system of health insurance as the main component in a reformed health service, the resulting reformation of the NHS along a purchaser-provider split of functions was both radical and comprehensive. It was, indeed, a Big Bang although the fuse might have been rather lengthy. The Government's management of this major shift in policy was accomplished after some bitter and public feuding with the British Medical Association and Royal College of General Practitioners but the policy was, indeed, implemented. More recently, attempts to revise GP and surgeon contracts provoked strong resistance from some sections of the medical profession.

The role of politicians both individually and corporately as managers has, perhaps, been understated. Their management perspective derives largely from a set of values which are then transformed into policies, sometimes with compromises having to be made along the way. The slogan that politics is the art of the possible has been reiterated by Lee & Mills (1985) who describe policy as having to reconcile what is politically feasible and technically desirable. There is, therefore, in the realm of political management a range of perspectives to be anticipated, considered and adjudicated in the light of ideological principles, economic circumstances and projections, political pragmatism and, at times, ethical demands.

Health care managers also need to have regard to multiple stakeholders' perceptions of what represents a good quality health service but in their case, more so than is the case with politicians in Government, they are likely to be subjected to evaluative criteria that are not necessarily of their own choosing. Do health care managers, then, have any autonomy or discretion in deciding between competing claims on resources? Are they able to make 'rational' decisions?

In 1995 the case of Child B, a ten-year-old girl suffering from acute myeloid leukaemia, highlighted the types of decisions that health care managers, in consultation with clinicians, have to make.

After a bone marrow transplant, the disease appeared to have been cured but the leukaemia returned and clinicians told the girl's father that she had only a few weeks to live. He contacted a private practitioner who was willing to treat Child B with a new treatment that would cost £75 000. The health authority refused to fund the treatment or provide a second bone marrow transplant since expert opinion was that the chances of success were extremely slim.

A high profile legal battle ensued and eventually the Court of Appeal found in favour of the health authority. An anonymous benefactor provided the funds for the treatment and the girl survived for another year before a further relapse led to her death. Although this particular example achieved national media attention,

> decisions involving ethical and cost-effective considera-
> tions, are at the heart of policies and local decision
> making that attempt to allocate resources according to
> the important criterion of cost-effectiveness.

Strategic choice

In their attempt to develop a theory of public management,
Ranson & Stewart (1994) refer to management as a process,
the starting point of which is 'strategic choice of priority
amongst purposes and the best means of achieving them'
(p. 33). This process of decision making rests on values, the
central box of the model set out in Figure 1.1 on p. 4 in
Chapter 1, and on the purposes and objectives of the organisation. They remark that 'strategic choice determines the
significant changes in direction which an organisation needs
to make in relation to a changing environment' (p. 34).

According to Ranson & Stewart, the process of determining strategic choice is dependent on a number of management
tasks. These are:

- policy planning
- staff motivation, communication and development
- organisational development
- relations with the public
- review and evaluation

It could, perhaps, be argued that management tasks are
themselves dependent on strategic choice since the overarching
aims of any organisation might change over time. No strategic or business plan remains or should remain intact for years
on end since different external circumstances such as new
legislation, new government policy, a shift in emphasis in
order to compete for commissioners or purchasers of services
will require adjustments to the organisation's policy and planning. Strategic choice, then, is driven not by the conventional
tasks of management but by the exigencies of the external
environment and this is markedly the case within organisations which are a constituent part of the NHS.

The need to respond to targets, for example, that are set by Government serve to limit strategic choice. Certainly, rational choice is confined, or, in Simons's terminology 'bounded', by the need to conform to the priorities laid down 'from above'. Managers within the health service are beginning to find an agenda already written for them by politicians and key policy drivers. For example, decisions communicated by NICE have to be implemented within three months. The discretion to make strategic choices based on values shared at all levels within, for example, a health care trust is becoming problematic. As a consequence, the criteria for evaluating not only individual trusts and primary care organisations but the NHS as a whole are in danger of being reduced to proxy indicators rooted in notions of economy and narrow interpretations of efficiency. Waiting lists, numbers on the list and length of waiting time for certain operations; clinical outcomes for operations compared across trusts; certain NSF targets: these are examples of the ways in which managerial and professional standards imposed traditionally from 'within' are being countermanded by numerical measures imposed from outside. Clinical governance, as Chapter 5 demonstrates, will continue to be a key component in the apparatus for monitoring and reviewing the quality of services. This prompts the question: what is meant by 'quality'?

Quality

Chapter 4 deals in some detail with the application of the term 'quality' to evaluating health care services. Here, we will be content with exploring the validity and applicability of this concept to the role of management within the health service context.

The term 'clinical governance' is essentially a comprehensive imperative to maintain, enhance and continuously review the quality of health care services. However, 'quality' as an agreed objective for all health service personnel, is both a useful and a deceptive word: useful because it emphasises the constant need to maintain high standards of services within the public domain; deceptive because its interpretation is elusive and dependent on the perspective of the particular stakeholder. For example, the quality of a service might be indisputable in terms of the professional manner in which it was delivered. A surgeon's proficiency in carrying out complex operations might be admired by peers as being of high quality. Yet the operation itself might be inappropriate when a less intrusive intervention could have produced an outcome of similar or longer-lasting benefit to the patient.

The authors of this book were commissioned by a Government department to undertake an evaluation of two major projects run over three years in order to prevent or delay the admission of vulnerable elderly people (some with dementia) to hospitals or residential care.

One of the evaluation criteria specified by the department was 'quality of service'. One particular event prompted the research team to rethink its mode of questioning on this criterion. Mrs Green (not her real name) was asked her opinion of the home care service that she was receiving on a two day a week arrangement. Her answer was that the person who provided this service was extremely helpful, did more than she was paid to do and that she was very pleased with the service.

The researcher then asked: 'If you could have only one kind of help (we deliberately avoided using the word "care" or "service") what would you choose?' She said that it would be someone to do her garden. When her husband was alive he did the gardening and the garden was their 'pride and joy'. She was arthritic; had no family living near or neighbours who might help. The sight of an overgrown patch made her feel sad.

Under the flexible multi-agency innovative approach that characterised this particular project, arrangements were made to hire a gardener. The home carer continued to provide a service.

This example highlights two potential difficulties in evaluating 'performance' in the public sector:

(1) There is an understandable tendency to use words that relate to the professional perspective: care, services, support. This then prescribes the choices offered to intended beneficiaries whereas the generic word 'help', in the context of health and social care, is not as limiting. In the case of Mrs Green, quality of service meant 'the kind of help that you would put as your first choice' i.e. what is the most appropriate help in terms of enhancing a sense of well-being?

(2) Outcomes of service are often multi-dimensional. We shall explore this statement in Chapter 5. In brief, a successful clinical outcome such as a hip replacement, improving the patient's mobility, could have serious financial consequences for a person who could wait no longer for the treatment as an NHS patient and who went to the private sector for the operation. There are many people like Mrs Green who value help not for its outcome in terms of the service's objectives, e.g. cleaning the house, or maintaining a tidy and clean environment, but in the outcome produced through the process of helping, such as having company, or feeling 'cared about'.

Health care managers are likely to be judged by interpretations of 'quality' that have very little to do with the process of management, as set out by Ranson & Stewart (1994) but which have much more to do with highly measurable performance indicators. In 2003, the UK Government introduced new primary care contracts for general medical services. GPs, as managers of primary care groups, agreed to accept a link between the level of fees and externally determined criteria of 'quality'.

We refer in more depth in the next chapter to the quantitative measures of quality, such as performance indicators. These always concentrate on efficiency and accountability (Martin & Kettner, 1996) and not on process and outcome criteria. They have their place in the repertoire of criteria that can be applied in order to assess the performance of professionals and organisations, such as hospitals, in which they work. The potential problem occurs when they are treated as surrogate indicators for the whole variety of health service functions.

As we noted in Chapter 1, Maxwell (1984) was one of the first health care commentators to draw up a list of attributes of health care services that constituted a quality service. These were accessibility, acceptability, appropriateness, effectiveness, efficiency and equity. The list is clearly open to challenge and its validity will depend on whether the six criteria form a core consensus of all relevant stakeholders in the NHS or whether they represent the perspective of only one or two key groups. For example, users of health care services are unlikely to be interested in broad questions of efficiency or equity and their interpretation of what constitutes effectiveness, appropriateness, acceptability and accessibility might differ from that of medical practitioners, health care managers and politicians (Phillips *et al.*, 1994). As Martin & Kettner (1996) have observed, 'quality – like beauty – lies in the eye of the beholder' (p. 42).

In the context of consumerism, for example, the final arbiters of what can be regarded as a 'quality' product or service are the customers. Could managers within the NHS act as advocates of this customer supremacy dimension for evaluating their own effectiveness? From a review of the literature Martin (1993) identified 15 generally recognised quality dimensions that applied to human service programmes in the USA. Some, such as 'assistance', 'courtesy' and 'empathy', draw attention to the importance of staff attitudes towards clients. The only dimensions contained in Maxwell's list are accessibility and effectiveness ('performance'). Additional items are:

- communication: information is provided in easily understandable language
- competency: staff possess the requisite knowledge and skills
- conformity: the service meets established criteria

- durability: the programmes performance or results do not dissipate quickly
- reliability: services are operated in a dependable and reliable manner with minimum variation through time or between clients (an element here of 'equity')
- responsiveness: service is timely
- security: services are provided in a setting free from risk or danger
- tangibles: the appearance of the facilities, equipment, personnel and published materials is appropriate

A list of 15 constituents of quality health care services does, indeed, suggest that quality is multi-dimensional. In order to reduce the list to a more indicative set of items, Zeithaml *et al.* (1990) identified five major quality dimensions of human service programmes. In rank order, with the weighting given alongside, these are:

(1) reliability   32
(2) responsiveness   22
(3) assurance   19
(4) empathy   16
(5) tangibles   11

Reliability refers to how consistently the expectations of clients are satisfied; responsiveness entails providing services with a minimum of waiting (Martin & Kettner, 1996).

Yet, all the five key attributes of 'quality' have been transformed into terms which many of the responding service users would not use. Therefore, even in a survey which seeks to canvass the views of patients and other service users, there is a danger that the researchers are interpreting the data according to their own notions of quality categories. For example, reliability could imply that service users are gratified when the health care professional, perhaps a district nurse or occupational therapist, turns up at the time and on the day that they agreed or that their appointment at the hospital was not cancelled. Attempts to classify dimensions of 'quality' are apt to become exercises in simplification. As Martin & Kettner argue, 'quality' as a concept is multi-dimensional but so are the individual dimensions which have been listed in various texts on aspects of quality in the health care services. As a further example, responsiveness might go beyond mere 'timeliness' and include people's perceptions of how well health care professionals listen and act upon patients' and family members' concerns and questions.

Given the complexity inherent in analysing what 'quality' means when applied to the health care system, it is perhaps appropriate to ask whether the use of the term is now anything more than a political mantra. Clinical governance, for example, puts quality at the heart of all medical and nursing activities. Clearly, managers within the health service have a responsibility to ensure that the organisation, be it a health care trust, primary care trust or local health board, maintains the very highest levels of professional competence. But Government policies continue to equate quality with measurable, 'objective' indicators that might say very little about reliability, responsiveness (apart from length of time on waiting lists), assurance or empathy.

Of course, it could be argued that political anxieties about waiting lists have been prompted by patient and media revelations about the plight, often of elderly people, who have waited many months, if not years, for treatment that would considerably improve their state of health. However, the Labour Government at the beginning of the twenty-first century seems preoccupied with prolonging the fallacy of its Conservative predecessors in its presumption that externally imposed targets, benchmarking and quasi league tables are the means of meeting public expectations of high quality services. Should, for example, local health boards or primary care trusts contract with the private sector to provide 'procedures' at higher cost now or make patients wait for 'cheaper' NHS provision and risk the possibility of a deterioration in health and the imposition of additional expenditure further down the line?

This is a problem for managers. If, as Government policies strongly suggest, the maintenance of high professional standards within the health service emanates not from the innate vocational dedication of doctors, nurses and allied professionals but from the imposition of yardsticks from above, it places managers in a difficult position. This is because they have to attempt to reconcile potentially competing interest groups' assessments of what contributes to or what defines high standards of health care. Inevitably, in the provision and consumption of health care services, there will be a plurality of interests and, consequently, a need for managers to develop some sort of evidence base for their own performance.

Differing perspectives

Any attempt to evaluate the 'success' of health care systems and specific elements within such systems requires a multi-perspective approach. For example, Smith & Cantley (1985) considered the many ways in which a psychogeriatric hospital's 'performance' could be assessed. It was, they argued, fallacious to assume that only output measures, such as numbers of operations, throughput of patients and staffing numbers, could adequately assess a hospital's status since it was multi-functional and, therefore, had to have regard to a number of objectives.

They sought the views of patients and their relatives and relatives' support groups and the views of the providers of services. Methodologically, they used a number of data sources and data collection methods (a strategy known as pluralistic evaluation) and made a tentative judgement about the success of hospital services based on a variety of criteria of what constituted 'success'. Their multi-perspective research design showed that organisations, programmes and projects can be successful in some ways and failures in others and why successes or failures occurred.

In adopting their particular approach to evaluation, Smith & Cantley dismiss traditional methods of service evaluation as too rationalistic in following the idealised model of policy making referred to previously in this chapter. In practice, they claim, policy making is very confused, while ambiguity and confusion of purpose are typical of most agencies. In hospitals and other organisations, objectives vary between and within significant groups. Goals of services are complex, multiple, conflicting. They are, indeed, say Smith & Cantley, variously interpreted, notoriously ambiguous and sometimes difficult to locate at all.

One of the difficulties, according to Smith & Cantley, in evaluating the success of hospitals and other complex organisations is a presumption of consensus: that the interest of the organisation as a whole is equated with the interests of senior managers.

The chair of a health trust asked the chief executive to provide evidence that they were part of a successful organisation. He was being assured in meetings that the trust was providing quality services but wanted to have some more objective evidence that this was so.

The CEO was asked to look at what other trusts were doing and how their trust compared with others. What kind of information would the officer have to provide in order to make a valid comparison?

Thomas & Palfrey (1996) have emphasised the need to encompass a diversity of stakeholders' views in trying to evaluate health care services. Politicians, managers, clinicians, non-clinical staff, patients and patients' families will view the performance of a hospital not by its entire entity as an organisation but according to how parts of it impact upon their interests and expectations. Managers, therefore, have to bear the responsibility for ensuring that these differing perspectives are taken into account in monitoring and reviewing the totality of the organisation's performance.

The recently created Commission for Health Audit and Improvement recognises the need to involve all such stakeholders in their assessment of hospitals. This would seem to be an enlightened approach to evaluating the 'quality' of a secondary or tertiary hospital but it would appear to run counter to political pressure to classify 'good' and 'inferior' hospitals by reference to more limited criteria. Problems for managers can arise when there appear to be tensions between, for example, budgetary criteria and more qualitative dimensions of what constitutes good practice. Patients are likely to rate process criteria such as attitudes of staff, flexible visiting times and a personal, caring approach by clinicians as more important than ward facilities or output and outcome criteria that would be the concern of managers and medical personnel.

It is also worth noting that heads of various directorates within a hospital, such as estates, human resources and supplies, will also have their own specialist interests and priorities which must be catered for amongst other claims upon the organisation's budget. Strategic health authorities and health care trusts also have to take into account demands for resources that arise from prescribing drugs and medication and, increasingly, projected claims for damages in the wake of alleged negligence. The complex nature of management tasks in the NHS suggests that textbook definitions of 'effective management' or 'models of good leadership' might be rather simplistic in their attempts to transpose ideas from the commercial world to the public sector. Similarly, we could ask whether it is appropriate to transfer methods of testing clinical efficacy to assessing the effectiveness of health care managers?

There is tangible evidence, for example, in accounting terms of over-prescribing among some GPs. Such budgetary items are easy to measure. Yet, in health care systems generally, other sources of waste might go unnoticed, such as the quantity of drugs acquired on prescription but never used – the problem of concordance or non-compliance. The cost of treatment is not simply the cost of drugs or medical and nursing time but has to take into account recovery times, incidence of side effects and their treatment, rates of delayed discharge, use of additional care resources and related administrative costs.

Evidence-based practice

In Chapter 5 we devote some space to dealing with evidence-based practice and policies. Here we wish to introduce the topic as, what was considered previously, a controversial approach to evaluating the outcomes of clinical interventions and to discuss whether this approach is applicable to an evaluative approach to health care management.

The origin of the movement towards evidence-based medicine is usually attributed to Cochrane (1972), who insisted that the gold standard for accumulating hard data was the randomised controlled trial. This has gained such approval in the past three decades that original opposition from medical practitioners such as Fowler (1997) has now largely dissipated. Appleby *et al.* (1995) produced a clear rationale for the application of this approach towards more rational decision making in the health service. They make the case that evidence-based medicine could result in many patients receiving better care and enjoying better health. Less directly, it could also encourage a more considered and evidence-based approach to management, priority setting and policy making.

Evidence-based medicine and health care has extended, through the more recent development of health technology assessment (HTA), to embrace all types of intervention under the term 'technology'. A succinct definition of HTA has been presented in the 2001 annual report from the Department of Health HTA Programme:

> HTA considers the effectiveness, appropriateness and cost of technologies used in the NHS. In this context, 'technologies' is not confined to new drugs or pieces of equipment. It covers any method used by those working in the health services to promote health, prevent and treat disease and improve rehabilitation and long term care.
>
> (p. 1)

The foundation for making clinical and resource allocation decisions is the systematic review. This research activity seeks to draw out from a comprehensive literature search a consensus in terms of research findings that relates to a particular treatment or intervention that works in terms of clinical efficacy. NICE relies on the data produced from systematic reviews and drug trials to determine its recommendations, with the added consideration derived from stringent costings, on which treatment is more cost effective than another.

So pervasive is this evidence-based policy in relation to professional decision making within the health care services that it has been taken as a model for other human services. The probation service has, in some areas, been active in developing a 'what works' approach to the various community and custodial sentences available to practitioners in the judicial system (Raynor *et al.*, 1994). Sheldon & Chilvers (2000) have mapped out a position paper on how to apply the same principles of evidence-based practice to the field of social work while Davies *et al.* (2000) have espoused the same approach to an evaluation of a range of public sector services.

The common factor in all of these arenas of public services is that the locus of evidence is the point of engagement between practitioner (surgeon, nurse, GP, probation officer, community worker, social worker) and the service user. This is because the capacity to control potentially confounding variables is quite promising in a situation where one course of action is implemented on an individual recipient. Complications in the process of sifting evidence in order to establish a cause-effect nexus can arise when the intended beneficiary could be not just the individual service receiver but the wider population. For example, rehabilitating offenders and preventing further crime is of clear benefit to society at large.

Where this direct contact between service provider and recipient is not present (as in the case of managers within the public sector) is there a case for attempting to evaluate their performance on the same basis of carefully researched evidence? Homa (1998) thinks that there is. He asserts that evidence-based management uses reliable information, based on research, as the foundation for management and policy formulation at all levels. It is, he claims, an ethical and professional obligation for those engaged in health care. The result is improved patient care: 'Managers have the same duty as clinicians to act according to the evidence provided by reliable information, based on good research' (p. 18).

Homa sets out a number of key questions that a management team adopting an evidence-based management approach could usefully ask:

- what is the problem that we are trying to solve?
- why are we trying to solve it?
- is it the right problem on available evidence?
- where is the evidence to support this?
- what is the quality of the evidence and what does it tell us about what we should do?
- is the evidence generalisable to our situation or is it specific to another setting?
- has this been tried elsewhere and what was the outcome?
- if we proceed with this proposal, how can we extract maximum learning and share this with colleagues attempting to address the same problem?
- what evidence will we use to measure success and over what period of time?
- is this more important than the least important management initiative currently under way – and should the two be substituted?

Encouraging health care managers to take on a more evaluative approach to their role can be achieved by enabling them to enrol on undergraduate and postgraduate courses that include management research. 'It is important', according to Homa, 'to create time for managers to be trained in research techniques and encourage them to apply these to contemporary management problems' (p. 21). Managers should also be able to reflect on and evaluate the quality of their decision making. This, says Homa, will contribute to an evaluative climate in which constructive challenge is positively encouraged. We endorse this exhortation by Homa that managers (like other professionals working within health care organisations) have a responsibility to engender and sustain an evaluative culture. In a public service that is continually battling with apparently infinite demand, the need to ground resource allocation and prioritising decisions in sound evidence would appear to be irrefutable.

The Audit Commission also has a role to play in determining the rationale for spending in certain areas of health care and not in others. Targets set by Government should, perhaps, also be open to challenge in a system that allows for greater openness in a dialogue between central, regional and local decision making bodies. In moving towards a more evaluative culture within the top managerial spheres of health care organisations, questions will need to be asked about the possible ways in which the randomised controlled trial technique applied in clinical trials can be applied in the field of management; or whether this particular means of generating evidence is appropriate in order to assess the impact of managers in the health service.

Testable assertions

Roberts (1996) and his colleagues set out to devise a means of putting statements about health services to the test. Assumptions about the efficacy of various treatments and interventions were, they argued, no more than assumptions unless they were capable of being translated into statements that were testable. Such activities as aspects of health visiting, alternative therapies and community mental health team interventions could become established by custom and practice rather than by dint of their proven effectiveness.

Their criteria for evaluating whether a statement was testable are these:

(1) does the intervention have a single component or are there multiple components?
(2) will the intervention be targeted at a single, well-defined population or multiple, poorly defined populations?
(3) is the intervention a single or multiple process?
(4) is the intended health benefit a single outcome or a multiplicity of outcomes?
(5) are the intended outcomes easy or difficult to measure?

Each criterion is to be judged as being 'fully met', 'partially met' or 'not met'. A statement is deemed to be untestable if one or more criteria are 'not met' or two or more are 'partially met'. They give examples. The statement: 'Streptokinase in the early management of myocardial infarction reduces mortality' is testable. In this case, all five criteria are fully

met. In contrast, the statement: 'Long-term outpatient management of patients with asthma improves their lung function',
is considered to be untestable because criteria (4) and (5) are
fully met, but numbers (1) and (3) are not met, and number
(2) is only partially met.

Roberts *et al.* concede that testable assertions are more
likely to be found in the acute sector while claims for the
clinical effectiveness of many community and social care
interventions are largely untestable by his instrument. He
concludes that the enduring problem for health care will
be not what to do about ineffective interventions, 'for EBC
(evidence-based care) will take care of these' (p. 33) but what
to do about treatments which embody an assertion of clinical
effectiveness which is untestable. This he defines as a political
and managerial, not a scientific problem.

It is not impossible to devise statements relating to community and social care contexts that are amenable to testing
in the way proposed by Roberts *et al.*, even in terms of clinical
effectiveness. It is not so much the location of where interventions take place but the nature of the intervention. For
example, patients can and do administer insulin injections
at home; community nurses and district nurses carry out
treatments in people's own homes. Assertions about these
interventions can be phrased in a form that can be tested by
applying Roberts' five criteria of testability.

The main limitation of the testable assertion method is
that it is a statement which relies on effectiveness viewed
from an exclusively clinical perspective. There is, therefore, a
danger of promoting the fallacy that clinical efficacy alone is
the yardstick against which to evaluate health care services.
This approach does, however, bring into focus the question
of how management as a function can be assessed. Within
the sphere of clinical interventions there is usually a clearly
defined intended outcome. But how could we apply this strict
evaluative method to palliative care or interventions appropriate in a hospice? Relief of pain comes to mind as one
clear objective. Many other processes, however, do not have
precisely defined intentions. Patient comfort, well-being,
emotional stability and peace of mind can best be assessed

by patients themselves. This might involve the use of patient surveys – a method of data collection which, unfortunately, tends to be done without reference to patients' ideas on which questions are the important ones to ask.

Summary

If clinicians are to be held more to account by calculations of the success rate of certain operations and GPs according to criteria of 'quality' in their medical and organisational competences, how can managers and those to whom they are accountable evaluate their performance? Can evaluation touchstones other than keeping within budgets, restraining over-prescribing, reducing waiting lists and waiting times be applied? What, in effect, constitutes 'good management'?

According to the criteria laid down by Roberts *et al.* (1996) managers will need to explain in the form of a testable statement what they understand by 'improving services'. However, as we have stated earlier, they are subject to conflicting demands because different stakeholders will define 'success' in different ways. In trusts, primary care organisations and in general practice managers will be judged by means of an array of measuring devices: benchmarking; audits; performance indicators; performance management; peer and external review; adherence to externally imposed targets; public pressure; media attention. They will be held to account by board members, senior civil servants, politicians and the public. They will, indeed, be required to adopt a pluralistic approach to assessing their adequacy and competence in attempting to achieve multiple targets and objectives. Performance management, which is the subject of the next chapter, is the framework in which this complex web of evaluative measures will have to fit.

References

Appleby, J., Walshe, K. & Ham, C. (1995) *Acting on the Evidence.* NAHAT Research Paper. National Association of Health Authorities & Trusts, Birmingham.

Caine, C. & Kenrick, M. (1997) 'The role of clinical directorate managers in facilitating evidence-based practice'. *Journal of Nursing Management*, **5**, 157–65.

Challis, L., Klein, R. & Webb, A. (1988) *Joint Approaches to Social Policy*. Cambridge University Press, Cambridge.

Cochrane, A. (1972) *Effectiveness and Efficiency: Random Reflections on Health Services*. Nuffield Provincial Hospitals Trust, London.

Crispin, P. (1996) 'Decisions, decisions'. *Journal of Management in Medicine*, **10** (6), 42–9.

Davies, H., Nuttley, S. & Smith, P. (2000) *What works? Evidence-based policy and practice in public services*. Policy Press, Bristol.

Department of Health (2001) *HTA Annual Report*. HMSO, London.

Detmer, D. (2000) 'Clinician-managers: the "boundary spanner" of the health service'. *Journal of Health Services Research and Policy*, **5** (4), Oct., 197–8.

Dixon, S., Booth, A. & Perrett, K. (1997) 'The application of evidence-based priority-setting in a district health authority'. *Journal of Public Health Medicine*, **19** (3), 307–12.

Dror, Y. (1989) *Design of Policy Sciences*. Elsevier, New York.

Etzioni, A. (1967) 'Mixed Scanning: a "third" approach to decision making'. *Public Administration Review*, (27), 385–92.

Farmer, J. & Chesson, R. (2001) 'Health care management: models for evidence-based practice'. *Journal of Management in Medicine*, **15** (4), 266–83.

Fowler, P.B.S. (1997) 'Evidence-based everything'. *Journal of Evaluation in Clinical Practice*, **3** (3), 239–43.

Haralambos, P. & Holborn, M. (1995) *Sociology: themes and perspectives*. Collins Educational, London.

Hewison, A. (1997) 'Evidence-based medicine: what about evidence-based management?' *Journal of Nursing Management*, **2**, 195–8.

Homa, P. (1998) 'What's your evidence?' *Health Management*, July, 18–19.

Johnstone, P. & Lacey, P. (2002) 'Are decisions by purchasers in an English health district evidence-based?' *Journal of Health Services Research and Policy*, **7** (3), July, 166–9.

Klein, R. (2000) 'From evidence-based medicine to evidence-based policy'. *Journal of Health Services Research and Policy*, **5** (2) April, 65–6.

Lee, K. & Mills, D. (1985) *Policy Making and Planning in the Health Sector*. Croom Helm, London.

Lindblom, C. (1959) 'The science of muddling through'. *Public Administration Review*, **19** (3), 517–26.

Martin, L.L. (1993) *Total Quality Management in human service organisations*. Sage, California.

Martin, L.L. & Kettner, P.M. (1996) *Measuring the Performance of Human Service Programs*. Sage, Calif.

Maxwell, R. (1984) 'Quality assessment in health care'. *British Medical Journal*, **288**, 166–203.

Morrison, R. (1995) 'Validation of nursing management diagnoses'. *Image – Journal of Nursing Scholarship*, **27** (4), 267–71.

Ovretveit, J. (1998) 'Medical managers can make research-based management decisions'. *Journal of Management in Medicine*, **12** (6), 391–7.

Phillips, C., Palfrey, C. & Thomas, P. (1994) *Evaluating Health and Social Care*. Macmillan, London.

Ranson, S. & Stewart, J. (1994) *Management for the Public Domain*. Macmillan, London.

Raynor, P., Smith, D. & Vanstone, M. (1994) *Effective Probation Practice*. Macmillan, London.

Roberts, C., Lewis, P., Crosby, D., Dunn, R. & Grundy, P. (1996) 'Prove it'. *Health Service Journal*, March, 32–3.

Sheldon, B. & Chilvers, R. (2000) *Evidence-based Social Care*. Russell House Publishing, Lyme Regis.

Simon, H. (1957) *Administrative Behavior*. Free Press, New York.

Smith, G. & Cantley, C. (1985) *Assessing health care: a study in organisational evaluation*. Open University Press, Buckingham.

Stewart, R. (1998) 'More art than science'. *Health Service Journal*, **108** (5597), 28–9.

Thomas, P. & Palfrey, C. (1996) 'Evaluation: stakeholder-focused criteria'. *Social Policy and Administration*, **30** (2), 125–42.

Vickers, G. (1965) *The Art of Judgement*. Chapman & Hall, London.

Zeithaml, V., Parasuraman, A. & Berry, L. (1990) *Delivering Quality Service*. Free Press, New York.

Chapter 4
Performance Management: Concepts and Approaches

In recent years increasing attention has been paid to the idea of 'performance management' within the NHS, as in most other fields of public sector services. The aim of this chapter is to define performance management and to disentangle the key elements of this approach to management within the health care sector. After defining performance management, we will turn to a number of approaches each of which has as its purpose the evaluation and improvement of service quality. The approaches are: performance indicators, best value, individual performance review and the quality movement. In various ways they emphasise different elements of the model which we introduced in Chapter 1. For example, some have, at least in the past, focused mainly on 'inputs' as with the early performance indicators, some on 'process' in the 'implementation' of policies and some on 'outputs' and 'outcomes' as in 'best value' analysis.

Background to performance management

In some important senses there is nothing new about performance management (PM). An essential part of 'planning and doing' has always concerned questions like 'how are we doing?' and 'are we on target?' Over many years the approaches to, and emphases on, such questions have altered and the language used has changed. But the essence of PM for managers remains.

A useful definition of PM is that provided by Armstrong & Baron:

A *strategic* and *integrated* approach to delivering sustained success to organisations by improving the *performance* of the people who work in them and by developing the capabilities of teams and individual contributors. [our italics]
(Armstrong & Baron, 1998; reproduced in Armstrong, 1999, p. 429)

However, one difficulty with this definition is that it contains concepts which require elaboration if we are to approach some common understanding of what PM is about. We need to consider the three concepts emphasised in the definition: *strategic*, *integrated* and *performance*.

Organisational decisions are commonly seen as *strategic* if they concern:

- the scope of the organisation's activities
- the organisation's environment (clients, customers, etc.)
- major resource implications
- the organisation's values and culture
- long term issues
- complexity ('big picture' issues)

(Johnson & Scholes, 1999)

The more a decision displays the above characteristics the more one is justified in regarding the decision as strategic in nature. Managers need to keep their eye on the big picture (the strategic issues), even when involved in relatively small scale operational tasks. This increases the chances of managers remaining aware of the reasons why they are doing what they are doing, and is why it is important for managers to retain a 'helicopter' frame of mind which enables them to see the wood for the trees even when working on individual trees (Handy, 1998). When health care managers are involved in the detail of an interdepartmental conflict, they need, as far as possible, to keep their eye on the broader vision – the purpose of the health care system and the health care needs of the public.

PM is an *integrated* policy in several senses, for example:

- vertical integration: linking organisational, team and individual objectives

- functional (or horizontal) integration: linking functional activities in different parts of the organisation, e.g. assessment of potential and actual needs/demands (marketing), providing services/goods to clients/customers, financial management and human resource management (HRM)
- integration of individual needs with those of the organisation as far as possible

(Armstrong, 1999, p. 430)

Performance can be a particularly difficult notion to clarify, partly because there are many criteria which are available to evaluate 'performance'. In Chapter 1 we characterised 'evaluation' as a process which is concerned with judging merit against some yardstick (Phillips *et al.*, 1994, p. 1). How can one judge the merit or 'quality' of a policy, service or organisation's performance? There are a number of criteria which can be used in making such judgements. The criteria, which comprise an expansion of Maxwell's framework to which we referred in Chapter 1, include:

- responsiveness (for example, in terms of speed, accuracy and helpfulness)
- equity/justice/fairness (for example, in terms of allocating resources according to the degree of need)
- equality (for example, in terms of equality of access, opportunity or outcome)
- effectiveness (the achievement of specified goals)
- efficiency and cost-effectiveness (maximising the benefit/cost ratio as far as possible)
- economy (for example, the reduction of spending as far as possible)
- accountability (ensuring that the location, direction and content of accountability are clear, together with the mechanisms of control)
- accessibility (for example, in terms of travel distances and waiting times for particular services)
- appropriateness (for example, ensuring that services are relevant to people's needs)
- acceptability (to all key stakeholders, including the intended beneficiaries, those who pay for the services and

the professionals, managers and politicians who plan and deliver the services)

- choice (for example, giving people reasonable choice as to which service provider to use)
- ethical considerations (for example, that services are provided in a way that satisfies established notions of ethics, such as beneficence and honesty)

The criteria are not mutually exclusive; sometimes the boundaries between them might be blurred; sometimes the criteria might overlap; for example, the acceptability of a service might depend on its responsiveness to users' needs and wishes. Furthermore, there is no a priori method of prioritising the criteria in terms of their relevant weightings. This is a political matter which we will address later in the book. These criteria are addressed in various ways throughout this book. They are all useful, but inevitably and inherently limited, as individual criteria for judging the performance of individuals and organisations.

It is not uncommon for PM to be seen as synonymous with staff appraisal or individual performance review (IPR) but these approaches tend to focus on the performance of individuals, albeit linked to an organisation's strategic aims. In many ways this emphasis on individual performance is too limiting. Regular evaluations of the performance of individuals is, of course, important and an essential element in an overall approach to performance management. However, PM implies something more systemic than IPR. In an effective PM system there are clear lines of 'accountability' within, and where necessary between, organisations, and an emphasis on a system's progress towards achieving its long-term and short-term aims and objectives. We shall return to the issue of accountability in Chapter 6.

In addition, IPR generally focuses on effectiveness as the main, or even sole, criterion for judging performance – often encapsulated in the need to be seen to be achieving 'SMART' objectives, that is objectives which are specific, measurable, achievable, relevant/realistic and timed. Our view of PM does not limit itself to effectiveness as the performance criterion.

All the twelve criteria listed above are likely to be used at some time or other when evaluating performance within a PM system.

Performance indicators

A widely used aspect of PM in recent years is the use of performance indicators (PIs). The NHS was one of the first public sector organisations in the UK to introduce a systematic package of PIs. A number of attempts were made to find useful performance indicators for the NHS in the early 1980s, and in 1982/3 a range of indicators was introduced on a trial basis in relation to acute services, maternity services, and services for the elderly, the mentally ill and the mentally handicapped, as well as for cross sectoral services (e.g. ambulance and laundry services and estate management). Examples of these early PIs in the NHS included:

(1) *Acute services*
    (a) activity indicators
        (i) immediate admission rate per 1 000 population served
        (ii) average length of stay
        (iii) annual throughput per bed
    (b) financial indicators
        (i) cost per day and per case by hospital and district (actual and expected)
        (ii) inpatient catering costs per inpatient day by hospital
    (c) manpower
        (i) percentage breakdown of nursing staff by registered; enrolled; learners; auxiliary nursing staff (for various hospital types)
        (ii) acute sector nursing staff – number of day cases and inpatient days

(2) *Cross sectoral indicators*
    (a) ambulance services

Financial

(i)   cost per 1 000 population served

(ii)   cost of management and supervision as a percentage of total cost

Manpower

Overtime costs as percentage total staff wages and salary costs for ambulance staff

(b) laundry services

laundry cost per 100 articles by laundry

(c) estate management indicators

(i)   land owned or occupied

(ii)   building area

(iii) disposable land as a percentage of all land

(Department of Health and
Social Security, 1983a)

The PI trials in the NHS arose largely out of criticisms made by the Public Accounts Committee (PAC), and on 22 January 1982, in a written answer to a Parliamentary question laid down by Mr Edward Du Cann, the Secretary of State (Mr Norman Fowler) said that a pilot scheme was to be conducted in one regional health authority (RHA) using indicators of performance in the delivery of health services. These would enable comparison to be made between districts, and so help Ministers and the regional chairman at their annual review meeting.

One object of the trial use of performance indicators in the pilot region (Northern) was to explore the grey area between clinical discretion and management responsibility. For example, a comparatively low throughput of patients could be due to professional practices that are beyond the scope of management action, but on the other hand it could be due to administrative bottlenecks.

In evidence to the PAC on 22 March 1982, Sir Kenneth Stowe (Permanent Secretary at the DHSS) confirmed that the Department had embarked on the pilot scheme in the Northern RHA but warned of the limitations. At present, he suggested, performance indicators enable us to ask questions (suggested by the indicators), but they do not give us definitive judgements (PAC, 1982, p. 35). A full set of PIs were published for 1981, in 1983 (DHSS, 1983b).

Right from the start the PIs focused mainly on inputs (resources) and activities as opposed to outcomes or the impact of services. 'The indicators are thus essentially service rather than population orientated; inward rather than outward looking' (Klein, 1982, p. 403). This has remained one of the serious technical and conceptual limitations of PIs. But the problems are not only technical and conceptual. They are also political. The use of performance indicators raises some important questions: Whose information is it? Who is monitoring whom? And for what purpose? Suspicion and scepticism remain throughout health care systems. Clinicians sometimes see PIs as the tools which managers are using to tighten the controls on professional autonomy, while managers might see PIs as undue and ill-informed attempts at central control by the Government. Our discussions with staff in the NHS in recent years suggest that when the PIs are used to construct league tables, some professionals and managers become even more uneasy. In many cases, staff are more supportive of PIs being used to track their changing performance over time rather than as a mechanism to construct crude league tables which are often seen as a way of comparing hospitals or individual clinicians and surgeons who, according to those who favour market solutions to performance problems, think ought to be 'competing' with each other.

PIs can be seen as:

- *Dials*   Such a PI would provide a precise measure of inputs, outputs and outcomes based on a clear understanding of what good and bad performance entails. One would be able to 'read off' performance by looking at the PI. Public sector organisations have very few (if any) of these.

- *Tin openers*   These are PIs that open cans of worms; they provide questions rather than answers. They are probably the most common kind of PIs in the public sector. For example, in the NHS a reduction in the average 'length of stay' in a particular specialty is not a safe guide to the 'quality' of a trust's efficient management if some patients are discharged too early.

- *Alarm bells* These are PIs that give warnings that things are beginning to go wrong. One wonders whether many of Harold Shipman's victims (patients of a GP jailed for serial murders in 2001) might have been saved if a more effective 'alarm bells' information system had been in place. The question also arises in the case of the children's deaths following heart surgery in Bristol in the 1990s. At the risk of inappropriately mixing the metaphors, 'whistle-blowers' have sometimes been tempted to sound the alarm bells if, for example, they believe that insufficient resources are being allocated to particular arenas of health care.

(Carter *et al.*, 1992)

It is generally recognised that before information can be used to make robust judgements about the performance of health care systems it needs to reveal what is happening in relation to outcomes; that is, what is the impact of the services provided? To gather information on outcomes is very difficult. For one thing there is the problem of causality (see Chapter 1). If increased expenditure on clinical services is in an attempt to increase average life expectancy, how safe is it to assume that any increase in life expectancy a few years down the line has been *caused* by the increased expenditure? That is, is the increased life expectancy an outcome of the increased expenditure or have other factors contributed to the improvement (for example: economic prosperity, diet, increased exercise, reductions in cigarette smoking and improved environmental and occupational conditions)? If the latter have contributed, what has been the relative contribution of each of the causal factors?

Attempts have been made to disentangle various causal factors (or independent variables), for example, in relation to coronary heart disease (CHD). CHD risk tables have been developed in order to try to assess the likelihood of an event occurring given specific patient profiles (for example, in relation to cigarette smoking, blood pressure readings, cholesterol levels and family history) (Rabindranath *et al.*, 2002). Another problematic question is: 'when is an outcome an outcome?' What appears to be an outcome from the point of view of one part of the system might be seen as merely a means to an end (for example, a longer term outcome) from someone else's viewpoint. One way to deal with this is to use the notion of 'interim outcomes' and not to claim that 'final' outcomes have been evaluated. Another approach is to identify who are the main clients (intended beneficiaries) of a service and regard any impacts on those groups (intended and unintended, positive and negative) as the service's 'outcomes'. The following case study concerns the problem of intended and unintended (and positive and negative) outcomes in the clinical area of post-operative nausea and vomiting (Tramèr, 2000).

Post-operative nausea and vomiting (PONV) is a common complication associated with anaesthesia and surgery. It can cause significant patient discomfort and, in out-patient procedures, may result in readmission or delay discharge and require the diversion of additional resources to deal with the problems. Drugs which reduce the incidence and frequency of PONV are available, but the decision of whether to utilise such drugs as a preventive strategy or as a form of treatment remain somewhat inconclusive. It has been suggested that it may be better to see who vomits and then treat. On the other hand, is it acceptable to wait and see if a patient vomits or becomes nauseated before starting a treatment? In addition, there is stronger evidence that all interventions increase the risk of harm compared with not using them. For instance, using propofol in children undergoing surgical squint repair with prophylactic anticholinergics means that on average one child will have a bradycardia due to the oculocardiac reflex before another child profits from its short-lived antiemetic efficacy.

PIs are also problematic because:

- they need to be based on accurate data: such data are not always available
- professional health care workers (doctors, nurses and other clinicians) commonly see themselves as being accountable to their peers, not to what they sometimes see as a set of dubious and managerially defined indicators imposed by Government agencies
- they are often ambiguous in meaning: for example, if one health care agency (A) employs one nurse for every 20 patients and another (B) employs one for every 25 patients, does this mean:
  - A is overstaffed?
  - B is understaffed?
  - B is more efficient than A?
  - A has a more complex case mix?
  - A has decided as a matter of policy to provide a higher level of nursing care?
- they might encourage tunnel vision and myopia (Smith, 1993) – an emphasis on the things which are easy to measure in the short term might discourage activities which have longer term implications, for example, training and development
- they often emphasise processes and procedures which might come to be seen as ends in themselves
- they might encourage 'game playing' (Smith, 1993) – people attempting to manage expectations of their future performance by keeping their present performance artificially low, thus keeping some 'slack' in the system for comfort
- people might indulge in creative accounting (for example, in the way in which overheads are allocated) (Smith, 1993)

Nevertheless PIs have remained a key part of the mechanisms used by Government to evaluate the performance of local agencies in the field. In 1999 the NHS Executive published guidance (NHS Executive, 1999b) about the sets of clinical indicators and high level performance indicators being made available for:

- setting standards nationally, for example, through the national service frameworks and the National Institute for Clinical Excellence (NICE)
- delivering high quality services locally, backed by a statutory duty of quality based on the concept of clinical governance, lifelong learning and professional regulation
- monitoring standards externally, including use of the indicators as part of a Performance Assessment Framework and with the Commission for Health Improvement (CHI); (the new Commission for Healthcare Audit and Inspection is scheduled to be fully operational as from April 2004)

Developmental work has been undertaken with the medical profession (in particular the Joint Consultants Committee of the British Medical Association (BMA)) in order to find ways of evaluating outcomes and not just inputs and activity levels. Steps have also been taken to test methods of using league tables to make explicit the performance ranking of individual hospitals and even individual surgeons, for example in relation to 'success rates' of heart operations. Clearly such comparisons are difficult to make in a valid and reliable way because some hospitals, being recognised as centres of excellence, are likely to attract many of the more complicated and difficult cases (see Chapter 1). One can never be sure that one is comparing like with like.

At an international level the World Health Organisation has also used league tables to assess certain aspects of the performance of member states according to a variety of indices. *The Word Health Report 2000* (WHO, 2000) publishes these tables in a variety of formats and is available on the WHO's website (www.who.int).

Within the UK, the *NHS Performance Assessment Framework* (NHS Executive, 1999a) and the associated *A First Class Service: Quality in the New NHS* (NHS Executive, 1999b) seek to provide a more balanced use of performance than the early sets of PIs. The framework sets out a range of six areas for evaluation:

- health improvement
- fair access to services

- effective delivery of appropriate healthcare
- efficiency
- the patient and carer experience
- the health outcomes of NHS care

Some of these criteria (for example, efficiency, effectiveness and fairness/equity) partly reflect the range of evaluation criteria set out earlier in this chapter.

The Government's intention is to develop the PI system so that it will be robust enough to provide useful data in relation to all six of these areas. This clearly represents a more balanced and outcome-oriented approach than the original PI packages in the early 1980s. However, only time will tell whether the developing framework will provide managers and health professionals with what they need for planning and delivering health services which meet the needs of an increasingly demanding public. There are still a number of areas which require further clarification in the six specified areas. For example, what counts as 'health improvement', and what does 'fairness' mean in relation to access to services? and are we sure we can reliably identify and assess the health outcomes of NHS care?

There is also some concern within the Audit Commission and elsewhere about the ways in which some health service managers might be tempted to 'misreport' data (for example, in relation to waiting lists), a practice which the NHS chief executive in 2003, Sir Nigel Crisp, has described as 'reprehensible and inexcusable' (*Guardian*, 5 March 2003, p. 10). Useful and up-to-date PI data for the NHS may be found on the Department of Health website (http://www.doh.gov.uk/indicat/nhsci.htm).

'Best value' and what followed

One of the means adopted for seeking to improve health service management in the 1980s and 1990s was the policy of compulsory competitive tendering (CCT). Health care agencies were compelled by the Conservative Government to adopt CCT in relation, in the first instance, to the 'hotel services' of catering, cleaning and laundry. The Labour Government had opposed the introduction of CCT and when they were returned to power in 1997 they promptly announced their intention to replace the policy with the notion of 'best value' (BV). The BV approach, introduced in 1999, applies mainly to local authorities (LAs) but it also affects health care agencies, particularly in relation to those services where they are expected to collaborate with local authorities, for example, services for those with learning difficulties, those with poor mental health and for the elderly.

At the outset there were two main parts to BV (Audit Commission, 2001, p. 4):

(1) LAs were expected to develop BV performance plans (BVPPs) to monitor and report on performance against national and locally defined standards and targets. The BVPP was intended to set out future priorities and targets for improvement.

(2) Fundamental BV reviews (BVRs) of all services were intended to identify what needed to be improved and how this was to be done. Each BVR was to be followed by an inspection by the Audit Commission Inspectorate. The inspectors were then to grade the service which has been reviewed on two dimensions:
   (a) How good is the service? (rated as excellent, good, fair or poor). Three 'key questions' are used to make this judgement:
      (i) Are the LA's aims clear and challenging?
      (ii) Does the service meet those aims?
      (iii) How does its performance compare?
   (b) What are the prospects for improvement? (rated as excellent, promising, uncertain or poor). Again there are three 'key questions':
      (i) Is the BVR likely to drive improvement?
      (ii) How good is the improvement plan?
      (iii) Will the LA deliver the improvement?

(Note: in 2001 the second judgement replaced a previous formula: 'Is the service likely to improve? – yes, probably, unlikely or no')

An important element was the expectation that the LA should adopt the 4 Cs approach:

- challenge: has the LA fundamentally challenged what it does?
- comparisons: has the LA made rigorous comparisons (with meaningful comparators) throughout the BVR?
- consultation: has the LA made good use of consultation (with all stakeholders)?
- competitiveness: how competitive is the LA's choice of procurement?

In the need to 'compare' performance, PIs continue to provide useful data as 'tin openers' (Carter *et al.*, 1992), that is pieces of information that prompt further questions about the performance in question. For example, best value performance indicator (BVPI) 166 sets out a checklist of environmental health, good practice examining issues such as the range of written enforcement policies which a local authority has in place. A local authority can then be scored, with the score being compared with average scores for other LAs. A useful website for BVPIs is at www.local-regions.odpm.gov.uk.

During 2001/2 the Audit Commission introduced a more varied range of inspections, for example, 'light touch' inspections, inspections that cut across several services and some 'corporate health' type inspections, to replace the 'one size fits all' approach which characterised the first year or two of 'best value'. In England the move is towards the development of comprehensive performance assessment (CPA) in which the evaluation of specific services is supplemented by a system of corporate assessment in which inspectors are expected to make judgements about a range of issues including, crucially, an organisation's capacity for improvement. The first results of the CPA approach were published in December 2002 in relation to English unitary authorities, metropolitan authorities and county councils. Each of the 150 local authorities assessed in the first batch was placed in one of five categories: excellent, good, fair, weak or poor.

In Wales, a different approach is being taken with the 'best value' approach evolving into the 'Wales Programme for Improvement' in which there is greater emphasis on self-assessment by local authorities and the development of improvement plans (replacing the original BVPPs) including the results of 'Whole Authority Assessments'.

Bovaird *et al.* (2002) have argued that evaluation approaches which seek to reduce measures to single aggregated scores (as with CPA and the Department of Health's introduction of star ratings for NHS trusts) tend to give insufficient emphasis to a range of more externally focused issues, such as quality of life outcomes and local governance matters, such as the involvement of communities in local decision making and the ethical conduct of organisations.

Best Value and CPA-style thinking can help managers and professionals to focus on important performance issues, but it can also be seen as a rather cumbersome and over bureaucratic approach which forces people to spend large amounts of time on analysing performance data. Even though it was awarded an excellent grading the chief executive of a London Borough Council has been reported as describing the exercise as 'unnecessary, inconsistent and demotivating' (*Guardian*, 12 December 2002).

In both England and Wales a number of changes are being piloted in relation to best value and its successors and it is too soon to judge the extent to which the developments will result in an improved 'evaluation system' generally, and for health related services in particular.

Benchmarking

One of the processes which many authorities undertake as a part of their BV reviews is that of benchmarking. However, benchmarking has a longer history than BV and many organisations have found comparisons with similar agencies constructive in seeking improved performance. The process of benchmarking is most useful if managers and professionals not only compare PIs between their organisations and others but also study over a period of time why the differences exist. As Wisniewski (2001) argues:

> Benchmarking is about more than simply comparing numerical levels of performance. . . . It is about understanding

why there are differences in performance between organisations, and this involves looking in detail at the way
services are delivered and managed and at the processes
involved in service delivery that lie behind the benchmark
measures of performance.

(p. 86)

Thus there are basically two types of benchmarking
(Wisniewski, 2001):

(1) Data benchmarking
     This is commonly based on published PIs and is best
     viewed as a starting point – much in the same way as
     Carter *et al.* (1992) viewed PIs as 'tin openers'.

(2) Process benchmarking
     This involves an examination of how and why things
     are done as they are and a continuous search for ways
     of improving performance by comparing processes with
     those adopted by similar organisations, especially those
     which are judged to be high performers or 'best-in-
     class'. Sometimes this is done by an organisation paying
     several visits to their benchmarking partners and under-
     taking careful assessments of alternative ways of imple-
     menting plans and delivering services. Where there are
     insufficient resources for such a detailed study, a 'quick
     and dirty' alternative could be a telephone conversation
     with selected people in a benchmarked organisation.
     However, organisations can become coy when asked to
     share information on working practices. To the extent
     that health care managers see themselves working in a
     competitive environment they could see process bench-
     marking as a kind of 'industrial espionage' in which an
     organisation may be suspected of 'stealing' ideas in
     order to improve its performance, for example, in relation
     to increasing levels of patient satisfaction or reducing
     waiting times. In principle this resistance to 'sharing'
     ideas is one of the potential disadvantages of compet-
     itive market approaches to health care, for example, in
     which primary care trusts may be encouraged to flex

their muscles in favouring one NHS trust over another as distinct from more 'collaborative' approaches.

A useful website for those seeking further help with processes of benchmarking may be found at: http://www.benchmarking.co.uk

Individual performance review/staff appraisal

Individual performance review/staff appraisal (IPR/SA) is a mechanism which many health care agencies use to cascade their PM system down to the level of the individual employee. Typically, the individual has a range of 'SMART' objectives against which their performance will be judged at regular, commonly annual, meetings with their manager.

Some see IPR/SA as synonymous with 'performance management' (for example, see Department for Education and Employment, 2000) but it is probably more useful to see IPR/SA as just one element of a PM system which may be more broadly viewed as an overall approach to evaluating and improving performance (see the definition of PM at the start of this chapter). IPR/SA can then be seen as a way in which PM is vertically integrated within the service so that individuals' objectives are consistent with those of the service as a whole.

It is common practice for IPR/SA interviews to take place between appraiser/reviewer and appraisee/reviewee annually, though in some organisations they take place more frequently. The interviews require careful preparation (agenda setting and agreeing what information will be needed etc.) and involve:

(1) assessment/measurement/evaluation of performance (including self-assessment)
(2) feedback
(3) positive reinforcement, including constructive criticism
(4) exchange of views
(5) agreement on action plans

(Armstrong, 1999, pp. 448–9)

There are many variations in the ways in which managers plan and implement IPR/SA systems: for example, should rating scales be used in an attempt to let people know where they stand, or are they a gross over-simplification of people's performance? To what extent, if at all, should managers seek evaluative feedback from their staff on a 360° basis as opposed to seeing IPR/SA as purely a top-down process? Despite the variations, IPR/SA systems all seek to provide systematic information on the performance of staff which can be seen as a part of the organisation's overall PM approach.

An aspect of IPR/SA that has generated considerable interest within the NHS is the use of personal development plans (PDPs). For example, as Fisher points out (1999, p. 182), in some health care professions, 'such as nursing, PDPs have become obligatory as part of the process of continuous professional development that practitioners have to undertake in order to maintain their professional registrations' (see also Jones & Fear, 1994; UKCC, 1996).

The PDP is a document and process that encourages employees to:

- undertake a systematic diagnosis of their development needs
- present their needs to the training managers and their line managers in a way that should get them the training resources they need
- keep a record of their learning achievements against their learning targets
- provide others with a systematic profile of their competences and achievements

(Fisher, 1999, pp. 181–2)

The existence of IPR/SA systems commonly assumes that it is the individual's 'line manager' who will be expected to hold the individual accountable or responsible for their performance. This becomes more blurred in the case of professionals (especially medical practitioners, who traditionally have enjoyed a great deal of status and autonomy) who might prefer to see themselves accountable to their patients or to peers.

A dramatic example of conflict between managers and medical staff took place in South Wales in 1995. An NHS trust ran into financial difficulties, partly because medical staff were able to resist the implementation of a plan to make them redundant and to transfer others to another trust when the service they were providing was to be transferred. In the battle that ensued – including a vote of no confidence in the Chairman of the Trust Board and the Chief Executive of the hospital, passed by the medical staff – the Chairman and the Chief Executive of the Trust were replaced.

(Harper, 1999, pp. 45–51)

The power of medical practitioners can also be seen in the process of medical audit. This is a 'peer accountability' process in which 'clinically significant events' (Marinker, 1990, p. 120) are the subject of 'systematic, critical analysis of the quality of the medical care' (Fisher, 1999, p. 184). Here the medics have, generally speaking, succeeded in keeping their non-medical management colleagues out of the loop.

In a statement published in 1993 a number of important health care professional organisations issued a consensus statement about the nature of clinical management which they defined as 'the explicit identification of the range of financial and other resources available to provide patient care and the assurance that these resources are utilised to greatest effect for the benefit of the individual patient and groups of patients' (BAMM, BMA, IHSM & RCN, 1993 p. 7). As Ong has pointed out (1998, p. 209) this definition appropriately focuses on the well established 'tension between a focus on individual patients (the professional perspective) and groups of patients (the managerial perspective)'. As a result, the effective implementation of IPR/SA systems for health care professionals is likely to remain problematic for the foreseeable future.

Whether or not the assessment of performance is of 'professionals', the process needs to be undertaken with sensitivity and in accordance with appropriate ethical principles. Winstanley & Stuart-Smith (1996) have suggested the following principles:

- *respect for the individual*: people should be treated as 'ends in themselves' and not merely as 'means to other ends'
- *mutual respect*: the parties involved in PM processes should respect each other's needs and preoccupations
- *procedural fairness*: the procedures incorporated in PM should be operated fairly to limit the adverse effect on individuals
- *transparency*: people affected by decisions emerging from the PM process should have the opportunity to scrutinise the basis on which decisions are made

These principles are consistent with those which we have discussed elsewhere in the context of the evaluation of public services generally (Palfrey & Thomas, 1996). We believe that without adherence to these principles, it is likely that a IPR/SA system will have more difficulty in sustaining the support of those whose performance is being appraised.

The use of IPR/SA systems remains problematic. This is partly the result of people feeling unconvinced that such 'managerialist' models are appropriate in situations where a degree of professional autonomy (especially clinical autonomy) is seen as a sine qua non of an effective health care system. Even where there is agreement (or at least an acceptance) that IPR/SA should proceed, there are often problems concerning the details. For example, are staff (both appraisers and appraisees) adequately trained and skilled at undertaking the process effectively and appropriately? And in what ways, if at all, should such systems be directly linked to reward systems? And to what extent does IPR/SA underemphasise some important performance criteria, such as equity and ethics, as opposed to the more easily measured criteria, such as meeting deadlines. Such issues continue to produce problems in the planning and implementation of 'evaluations' at the level of individual members of staff. Many people remain uncertain about the question of whether IPR/SA systems lead to improved organisational performance (Leopold *et al.*, 1999, p. 188).

The quality movement

The notion of 'quality' has a long history in management and we have drawn attention to its often problematic interpretation in Chapter 3. For decades, industry used methods of 'quality control' to check that the products being delivered to customers were of acceptable standard. More recently, wider approaches to quality have been used, for example, quality assurance, quality circles, 'total quality management' and a range of accreditation schemes such as ISO 9000, Chartermark, and Investors in People (schemes in which organisations are seen by some to be 'badge collecting').

'Total quality management' (TQM) and related approaches have been taken up by many organisations in the last 20 years or so. TQM is thought by some to represent a radical change in that it seeks to alter the organisation's *culture*, with an emphasis on a widespread *commitment* to get things *right first time* and to tailor the services/goods provided to match the customers' (*internal and external customers*) wishes/needs (Crosby, 1979; Koch, 1991; Ellis & Whittington, 1993; Morgan & Murgatroyd, 1994), though some remain more sceptical about many aspects of the 'quality industry' (Kirkpatrick & Martinez Lucio, 1995; Pfeffer & Coote, 1991).

Although one should be appropriately sceptical about how desirable and realistic 'quality' prescriptions are, such concepts can offer useful, albeit limited frameworks for evaluating the processes, outputs and outcomes of organisations. One of the popular approaches to assessing and improving quality in organisations is ISO 9000 (formerly British Standard 5750) certification by a body accredited under the auspices of the United Kingdom Acreditation Service. Advocates of this approach point to its rigorous and systematic mechanisms. On the other hand, it can be argued that the approach concentrates on requiring organisations to set their *own* standards and to measure the extent to which effective *procedures* are in place to achieve those standards. The approach does not necessarily require the achievement of 'high' standards of service.

An alternative approach to assessing and improving quality is to rely on institutional mechanisms. Examples include the Audit Commission, the Commission for Healthcare Audit and Inspection (CHAI), community health councils (which are to continue in Wales) and a range of commissioners or 'ombudsmen' relating to local government, central government and the health service. These various bodies commonly identify specific problems with health services and develop ideas as to how the problems should best be dealt with. To this extent the institutions can be an aid in evaluation, both in the collection and analysis of data and in discussions about the evaluative criteria which, in the institutions' views, should be used in carrying out the evaluations.

In an overview of TQM in the public sector, Morgan & Murgatroyd (1994) identify ten key principles which service providers need to take into account:

(1) *customer-driven services*: a focus on providing outstanding service at an appropriate cost to all primary customers

(2) *strategic focus on outcomes and processes*: TQM is a focused practice that seeks to turn strategic intent into direct, practical achievement

(3) *driven by goals and values, not regulations*: staff working in the public sector should be able to make decisions on the basis of clear processes which are value-driven rather than regulatory and disabling

(4) *empowering for communities, workers and customers*: the aim is to empower people to achieve that which they need and to achieve it by working cooperatively and creatively

(5) *effective and efficient*: TQM is a set of management practices which aim to improve performance and increase customer satisfaction while lowering costs

(6) *evaluated as successful by customers in comparison with comparative providers of services*: when customers compare the performance of a public service with that of

others or with private sector provision, they will recognise value for money and quality performance in what they see

(7) *valued by staff and customers alike*: there will be a respect for process and service quality among everybody associated with the service

(8) *enterprising, not simply spending-oriented*: TQM encourages the public sector both to reduce costs and to gain income from being more enterprising about the potential resale of processes, technology, ideas, resources, etc: teams should be encouraged to be entrepreneurial, not just spending oriented

(9) *proactive rather than reactive*: TQM encourages teams and management to anticipate and plan before they act – it seeks to encourage insightful forecasting, planning and the management of development

(10) *benchmarked against the best in the world*: the aim of every public sector organisation should be to lead the world in the provision of its core services in terms of customer satisfaction, efficiency and appropriate cost: careful benchmarking will enable them to show the extent to which they can deliver to this promise

Morgan & Murgatroyd (1994) also offer a list of determinants of customers' perceptions of quality in service provision:

- reliability: e.g. is the service performed at the designated time?
- responsiveness: e.g. willingness to provide the service
- competence: e.g. possession of the required skills and knowledge to perform the service
- access: approachability and ease of contact with the providing institutions
- courtesy: e.g. politeness, respect, and friendliness of contact
- communication: e.g. keeping people informed in language they understand; also listening to them; explaining the service, options and cost; assuring people that their problems will be handled

- credibility: e.g. belief that the providers have the person's best interests at heart; trustworthiness and honesty
- security: e.g. freedom from danger, risk or doubt
- understanding/knowing the individual: e.g. making the effort to understand one's needs by providing individualised attention
- appearance/presentation: e.g. the physical facilities, appearance of personnel, equipment used, etc.

Morgan & Murgatroyd's principles provide a framework for evaluating certain aspects of policies and public sector services. It could be argued that the notion of 'quality' encompasses all (or at least most) of the other evaluation criteria. Certainly some of them (for example, effectiveness and efficiency) are explicitly included in Morgan & Murgatroyd's 'checklists'.

The criteria included in most notions of TQM tend to place much greater emphasis on customer satisfaction and the reduction of waste than on some of the wider criteria such as appropriateness (as defined by professionals), equity and equality. 'Quality' in the business management sense is thus often seen by managers and their trainers in a rather narrow way. Furthermore, the 'quality management' literature tends to be prescriptive and 'top-down' in approach. There is relatively little rigorous research on the ways in which 'quality' initiatives help public sector organisations to evaluate and improve their services. Nevertheless, the quality movement continues to be influential within the NHS as a framework within which professionals and their managers seek to evaluate and improve performance.

However, others have displayed a greater degree of scepticism about TQM approaches. For example, Kirkpatrick & Martinez Lucio (1995) have identified a number of limitations and problems of TQM in the public sector. In particular, quality can be seen as a means of increasing managerial control over 'professionals' (e.g. doctors and nurses). A part of this process involves the use of the notion of quality as a means of legitimising managerial changes which are *claimed* to be in the interests of customers.

Second, quality is often defined narrowly (e.g. 'value for money', conformance to standards or fitness for purpose), but there is often conflict between different aspects of 'quality' (e.g. 'better' services versus cost containment). The notion of 'quality' is thus problematic. Third, it is often claimed that quality initiatives improve arrangements for people in relation to 'exit' and/or 'voice' (Hirschman, 1971). The former notion implies an ability to easily withdraw from one service provider and to choose to go elsewhere for a better service, thus putting pressure on every provider to ensure that its services are satisfactory to the customers. The notion of 'voice', on the other hand, represents the ability that people (service users and the public at large) might have to influence the development of the services – 'empowerment' in the modern parlance.

There are, however, serious limits involved with the concepts of exit and voice. Exit (or choice) is often not possible for the intended beneficiaries of services. 'Purchasers', commissioners, or the 'client' side of contractual relationships might have some choice concerning which providers or contractors to use, but individual members of the public are less well placed. In the case of voice, is there real empowerment for people (e.g. user involvement in the prioritising of services) or is it just a matter of having statements in documents (mission statements, policy documents, etc.)? Is 'getting close to the customer' just rhetoric? In practice, there is often little user/community involvement in key decision making, although there have been various attempts to use neighbourhood groups, locality planning teams, citizens' panels and juries, and similar mechanisms, in some regions.

Another sceptical strand in the literature on quality is that developed by Pfeffer & Coote (1991), who view most established quality approaches as having too narrow a focus because they do not adequately acknowledge important distinctions between commerce and welfare. The authors propose an alternative model, a democratic approach, which recognises that 'the public has a complex set of relationships with welfare services, not just as customers, but as citizens and providers too' (1991, p. 1). This model of 'quality' gives more attention than most established models to the purpose of public services, responsiveness, giving the public more power and participation, equity and rights.

In 1999, the Government set out its framework for quality improvement and fair access in the NHS (NHS Executive, 1999b), the main elements of which include:

(1) clear national standards for services and treatments through national service frameworks (NSFs) to tackle unacceptable variations in quality across the country, and the (then) new National Institute for Clinical Excellence; the emphasis here was on 'evidence-based' guidance, with NICE assessing new and existing interventions for their clinical and cost-effectiveness

(2) local delivery of high quality health care, through clinical governance, underpinned by modernised professional self-regulation and extended lifelong learning for continuous updating of skills and knowledge

(3) effective monitoring of progress through agencies and mechanisms such as the Commission for Health Improvement (CHI), intended to integrate a number of evaluation functions including the health value for money work of the Audit Commission and a new NHS performance assessment framework (NHS Executive, 1999a)

At the time of writing these arrangements are not yet all in place. How effective they will be in promoting high quality health care will be a fruitful area for research in the next few years.

Another approach to enhancing quality, which has gained ground in recent years, is the 'business excellence model' developed by the European Foundation for Quality Management. The model comprises two sets of variables – enablers and results – and, in essence, suggests that if it is possible to get the enablers right it will significantly increase the chances of attaining the required results.

The enablers

- leadership
- people management
- policy and strategy
- resources
- processes

Results

- people satisfaction
- customer satisfaction
- impact on society
- business results

Some work has been done utilising the model in the context of health care agencies (see, for example, Freer & Jackson, 1998) and further developmental work has been done in order to increase the relevance of the model to the public sector. Although the excellence model has attracted a good deal of attention in recent years, it is too soon to judge its usefulness compared with alternative approaches to evaluating and improving quality of services.

Summary

What do health care managers and others need to learn from the approaches analysed in this chapter? They clearly need to be aware of the changing nature of the performance management and evaluation debates as they continue to unfold and to develop their ability to plan and undertake appropriate evaluations of their organisations' performance.

In 1985 a critical analysis of some of the key problems in evaluating performance in health care systems (Scrivens *et al.*, 1985) included a review of the criteria used to select measures for evaluating health interventions. Much of the debate centred around the meaningfulness and usefulness of various approaches to what we now call performance management. The discussion was further developed by Flynn (1986) who analysed the problems of assessing outcomes and of ambiguous and conflicting objectives. One suggested solution was that 'the inability to demonstrate the effectiveness of a whole service should not deter managers from trying to determine the relative effectiveness of parts of the service' (Flynn, 1986, p. 398). In this sense the more specific a goal is (for example, 'to help the patient to become competent and confident in administering' a particular self-treatment as opposed to a goal that says 'to create a healthier population') the easier it usually is to demonstrate whether the desired outcome has been achieved.

There is increasing emphasis on outcome measures not only in the NHS but in the public sector generally. This is reflected in a report published by the National Audit Office (NAO) in 2001. Public service agreements (PSAs) now set out what the Government aims to achieve.

> Each PSA includes the aim of the Department or policy area, supporting objectives and related performance targets which underlie the resources allocated to them in public expenditure reviews. Service delivery agreements have now also been introduced which specify how these targets will be achieved.
>
> (NAO, 2001, p. 1)

The report also points out that the PSA targets are:

> more orientated towards the specification of desired outcomes for public services, such as improved health and life expectancy, rather than outputs of Departmental activities, such as the number of operations, or processes or inputs. The percentage of PSA targets that address outcomes increased from 15% in 1999/2000 to 68% for 2001/4.
>
> (NAO, 2001, p. 1)

One of the difficult problems that has to be faced in designing meaningful outcome measures is that in many public services the intended outcomes cannot be achieved by one organisation working in isolation. In research carried out by the NAO, 75% of departments said that 'they faced a great challenge in agreeing outcome measures which are shared or influenced by others' (NAO, 2001, p. 2). The prescriptions in recent years to plan and deliver services in a more 'joined-up' way are laudable but difficult to achieve in practice. The problems of achieving effective collaboration between different public sector agencies are well recognised (for example, see Booth, 1981; Challis *et al.*, 1988; Huxham, 2000) but there are, as yet, no demonstrably robust prescriptive models on how to achieve the necessary degree of 'joined-upness' (Hudson *et al.*, 1999).

Another vexed question is the burden that data collection and analysis can place on professionals and managers. Anecdotal evidence suggests that there is a considerable degree of resentment among service planners and deliverers about what is often seen as the 'extra' work of collating data for external inspection agencies. Neither are all professionals and managers convinced about the validity and reliability of the data used in performance indicators, league tables and other evaluative mechanisms.

The debate about what forms PM should take continue. Few would deny that it is important for the performance of health care agencies to be evaluated on a systematic basis. What remains a widely contested question is what are the most appropriate and effective means of achieving this. It is possible that a reduction in the number of targets that are imposed on health care agencies has a role to play. There is no 'one way forward', but there is a need for primary care trusts and NHS trusts to be allowed a degree of autonomy in selecting their own high priority objectives (the top right hand box of the model outlined in Figure 1.1 on page 4 Chapter 1) within the overall strategic guidance from Strategic Health Authorities and others. External imposition of large number of detailed targets may be well intentioned but it can also be counter-productive.

References

Armstrong, M. (1999) *A Handbook of Human Resource Management Practice*. Kogan Page, London.

Armstrong, M. & Baron, A. (1998) *Performance Management: the new realities*. Institute of Personnel and Development, London.

Audit Commission (1991) *Report and Accounts.* HMSO, London.

Audit Commission (1996) *By Accident or Design: Improving Accident and Emergency Services in England and Wales.* HMSO, London.

Audit Commission (2001) *Changing Gear: best value annual statement 2001.* Audit Commission, London.

Baggott, R. (1998) *Health and Health Care in Britain.* Macmillan, London.

BAMM, BMA, IHSM & RCN (1993) *Managing Clinical Services: a consensus statement of principles for effective clinical management.* BAMM, BMA, IHSM & RCN, Stockport and London.

Black, N. (1998) 'Clinical governance: fine words or actions?' *British Medical Journal,* **326**, 297–8.

Booth, T. (1981) 'Collaboration between the health and social services'. *Policy and Politics,* **9** (1), 23–49 and (2), 205–226.

Bovaird, T., Loeffler, E. & Martin, J. (2002) 'From corporate governance to local governance: stakeholder-driven community score-cards for UK local agencies?' Paper presented at the Annual Conference of the British Academy of Management, London.

Carter, N., Klein, R. & Day, P. (1992) *How Organisations Measure Success: The Use of Performance Indicators in Government.* Routledge, London.

Challis, L., Fuller, S., Henwood, M., Klein, R., Plowden, W., Webb, A., Whittingham, P. & Wistow, G. (1988) *Joint Approaches to Social Policy.* Cambridge University Press, Cambridge.

Crosby, P. (1979) *Quality is Free.* McGraw-Hill, London.

Davies, H., Nutley, S. & Smith, P. (2000) *What Works? Evidence-based policy and practice in public services.* Policy Press, Bristol.

Davies, H. & Nutley, S. (2000) 'Healthcare: evidence to the fore', cited in Davies, Nutley & Smith (2000).

Department for Education and Employment (2000) *Performance Management in Schools.* HMSO, London.

Department of Health (1998) *A First Class Service.* HMSO, London.

Department of Health (1999) *Clinical Governance: quality in the new NHS* (Circular HC 1999/065). HMSO, London.

Department of Health and Social Security (1983a) *Health Care and its Costs.* HMSO, London.

Department of Health and Social Security (1983b) *Performance Indicators. National Summary for 1981.* HMSO, London.

Ellis, R. & Whittington, D. (1993) *Quality Assurance in Health Care: a Handbook.* Edward Arnold, London.

Fisher, C. (1999) 'Performance Management and Performing Management', cited in Leopold, Harris & Watson (1999).

Flynn, N. (1986) 'Performance measurement in public sector services'. *Policy and Politics,* **14** (3), 389–404.

Freer, J. & Jackson, S. (1998) 'Using the business excellence model to effectively manage change within clinical support services'. *Health Manpower Management,* **24** (2), 76–81.

Guardian 12 December 2002.

Guardian 5 March 2003.

Handy, C. (1998) *Understanding Organisations*. Penguin, Harmondworth.

Harper, G. (1999) 'The economics of the Scottish acute care hospital sector, 1991–94' (unpublished PhD thesis), University of Wales College, Newport.

Hirschman, A. (1971) *Exit, Voice and Loyalty: Responses to Decline of Firms, Organisations and States*. Harvard University Press, Massachusetts.

Hudson, B., Hardy, B., Henwood, M. & Wistow, G. (1999) 'In Pursuit of Inter-Agency Collaboration in the Public Sector'. *Public Management*, **1** (2), 235–60.

Huxham, C. (2000) 'The Challenge of Collaborative Governance'. *Public Management*, **2** (3), 337–57.

Johnson, G. & Scholes, K. (1999) *Exploring Corporate Strategy*. Prentice Hall, London.

Johnson, G. & Scholes, K. (2001) *Exploring Public Sector Strategy*. Prentice Hall, London.

Jones, N. & Fear, N. (1994) 'Continuing professional development: perspectives from human resource professionals'. *Personnel Review*, **23** (8), 48–61.

Kirkpatrick, I. & Martinez Lucio, M. (1995) *The Politics of Quality in the Public Sector: the management of change*. Routledge, London.

Klein, R. (1982) 'Performance, Evaluation and the NHS: A case study in conceptual perplexity and organisational complexity'. *Public Administration*, **60**, (Winter 1982), 385–407.

Koch, H. (1991) *Total Quality Management in Health Care*. Longman, London.

Leopold, J., Harris, L. & Watson, T. (1999) *Strategic Human Resourcing: Principles, Perspectives and Practices*. Financial Times Management, London.

Marinker, M. (1990) *Medical Audit and General Practice*. British Medical Association, London.

Maxwell, R. (1984) 'Quality Assessment in Health'. *British Medical Journal*, **288**, 166–203.

Morgan, C. & Murgatroyd, S. (1994) *Total Quality Management in the Public Sector*. Open University, Milton Keynes.

National Audit Office (2001) *Measuring the Performance of Government Departments*. HMSO, London.

NHS Executive (1999a) *The NHS Performance Assessment Framework*. NHSE, Leeds.

NHS Executive (1999b) *A First Class Service: Quality in the New NHS*. NHSE, Leeds.

Ong, B. (1998) 'Evolving perceptions of Clinical Management in Acute Hospitals in England'. *British Journal of Management*, **9**, 199–210.

Palfrey, C. & Thomas, P. (1996) 'Ethical Issues in Policy Evaluation'. *Policy and Politics*, **24** (3), July 1996, 277–85.

Pfeffer, N. & Coote, A. (1991) *Is Quality Good For You?* Institute for Public Policy Research, London.

Phillips, C., Palfrey, C. & Thomas, P. (1994) *Evaluating Health and Social Care*. Macmillan, London.

Public Accounts Committee (1982) *Seventeenth Report from the Public Accounts Committee*, Session 1981/82, May. HMSO, London.

Rabindranath, K., Anderson, N., Gama, R. & Holland, M. (2002) 'Comparative evaluation of the new Sheffield table and the modified joint British societies coronary risk prediction chart against a laboratory based risk score calculation'. *Postgraduate Medical Journal*, **78** (919), 269–72.

Scrivens, E., Cuningham, D., Charlton, J. & Holland, W. (1985) 'Measuring the impact of health interventions: a review of available instruments'. *Effective Health Care*, **2** (6), 247–60.

Smith, P. (1993) 'Outcome-related performance indicators and organisational control in the public sector'. *British Journal of Management*, **4**, 135–51.

Tramèr, M. (2000) Systematic reviews in PONV therapy. In: *Evidence based resource in anaesthesia and analgesia* (ed. Tramèr, M.). BMJ Books, London.

United Kingdom Central Council for Nursing. Midwives and Health Visitors (1996) 'PREP: you and your guide to profiling'. *Register*, **17**, Summer.

Winstanley, D. & Stuart-Smith, K. (1996) 'Policing Performance: the ethics of performance management'. *Personnel Review*, Summer, 66–84.

Wisniewski, M. (2001) 'Measuring up to the best: a manager's guide to benchmarking', cited in Johnson & Scholes (2001).

World Health Organisation (2001) *The World Health Report 2000: Health Systems: Improving Performance*. WHO, Geneva.

Websites: http://www.doh.gov.uk/indicat/nhsci.htm
http://www.doh.gov.uk/pricare/clingov.htm
http://www.benchmarking.co.uk
http://www.who.int
http://www.local-regions.odpm.gov.uk.

Chapter 5
The Evidence-based Organisation

The struggle to generate appropriate and effective means to evaluate the performance of health care agencies is compounded by the complexities of health care systems themselves. For example, one of the major external factors impinging on health care systems, depicted in the analytical framework model described in Chapter 1, is what has been termed the 'health care dilemma' (Phillips, 1997; Phillips & Prowle, 1992). The nature of this dilemma, which confronts virtually all health care systems, is depicted in Figure 5.1 below. It is a microcosm of the basic economic problem which confronts all individuals, organisations and societies – that of reconciling infinite wants, needs and demands with finite resource availability, in terms of income, time, expertise, and so on. As individuals, we have to choose how to allocate our income among competing demands; we have to decide how we will apportion our time among work, family and other

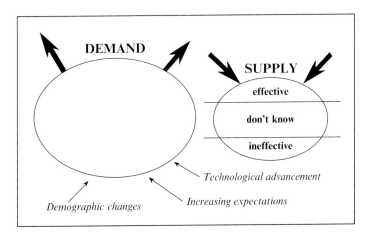

Figure 5.1   The health care dilemma

commitments and so on. The same issues apply to whichever unit one wishes to consider and health care systems are no exception.

The exponential increase in demand for health care services (depicted by the arrows from the demand ellipse in Figure 5.1) is occurring at the same time as pressures on governments and funding agencies to carefully manage the volume of resources available for health care services (depicted by arrows moving towards the supply ellipse).

The ever-increasing demands placed on health care services, despite general improvements in the health status of communities, is common across most health care systems. The factors contributing to these increases in demand are many but chief among them are:

- Demographic changes: people are living longer and there is a direct relationship between age and utilisation of health care services. Birth rates are lower than in previous generations and the proportion of elderly people within society is therefore increasing, which places even greater demands on available resources.

- Technological advancements: medical science and computer technology have advanced dramatically over recent decades, resulting in the development of new techniques and procedures, which have major implications for the delivery of patient care, for example, the developments in laser surgery, which have resulted in a shift to day-case procedures, speedier rehabilitation periods and time returning to normal functioning.

- Increasing expectations: diseases which would have resulted in death or severe debilitation are now treatable and, in many cases, preventable owing to the advancements in knowledge and changing practices. Accompanying these trends has been a change in people's expectations that health care services can meet a greater proportion of our needs; for example, anecdotes of patients taking information, downloaded from the Internet, relating to their particular condition, to their general practitioner, and requesting the recommended treatment are increasing.

The constraints in the supply of resources available for health care services are compounded by the fact that a percentage of interventions are known to work effectively, a percentage are known not to work, while it is not known whether the remainder of interventions work or not. What is also unknown is the actual percentage each category represents. For example, it has been estimated that up to 25% of all health services currently provided may be unnecessary (Borowitz & Sheldon, 1993); while 10–15% of health care interventions are known to generate health gain; and a similar percentage are known to reduce health status (Warner & Evans, 1993).

Debates on the topic of additional resources required to secure appropriate funding levels for health care services are clouded by issues relating to, for example, the effectiveness of interventions, the competence of health care professionals and the safety of health care facilities. The need for evidence on the effectiveness of interventions has resulted in something of an evangelistic campaign, over the past ten years or so, to ensure that clinical decisions are based on evidence as to what works and what does not work. In addition, the social status of doctors in society has shifted from that of expert, whose judgement was to be trusted and who were left to carry out their duties relatively unchallenged at the beginning of the twentieth century, to the current situation, where levels of public trust have been diluted as a result of high profile media cases, but also as an increasingly educated, informed and questioning public has sought reassurance that public finances were being used efficiently (Davies *et al.*, 2000a).

The nature of the health care dilemma, with ever increasing demands placed on health care services against constraints on the resources available to meet them, continues to be a major issue for those at all levels of policy making, decision making, commissioning services and the provision and delivery of health care services. The need to ensure that limited resources are channelled into effective interventions has provided additional impetus for managers and health care professionals to the drive towards evidence-based practice. It has been forcibly argued that, '. . . in the twenty-first century, the health care decision maker, that is anyone who makes decisions about groups of patients or populations, will have to practise evidence-based decision making' (Gray, 1997). Evidence-based decision making, according to Gray, is the ability to do the right things right. He catalogues the evolution of evidence-based health care (EBHC), in the UK context, from the period during the 1970s when economic pressures initiated an era when cost issues became significant factors for health care decision makers ('doing things cheaper'), through the quality initiatives of the 1980s ('doing things better') to the period when these were combined into the era of 'doing things right'. He provides a framework (based around focusing on interventions which do good, stopping those which do harm and developing research to assess the effectiveness of those whose effect is unknown) for its influence 'not only on how clinicians practise, but what they practise' (p. 22).

Foundations of evidence-based decision making

There are three characteristics that mark the evidence-based organisation (EBO) according to Gray (1997). First, the culture of such an organisation is dominated by an obsession with finding, appraising and using research-based knowledge in decision making. Second, in an EBO there will be systems for managing knowledge and for developing the skills of the individuals who work in the organisation. Third, the structure of an EBO should promote and facilitate evidence-based decision making. These characteristics and their relationship to the analytical systems model depicted in Chapter 1 are shown in Figure 5.2.

The principles of evidence-based decision making and EBHC are largely dependent on those associated with the notions of evidence-based medicine (EBM), although as we shall see later there are other factors that also need to be considered.

The philosophical origins of EBM can be traced back to the nineteenth century (Sackett *et al.*, 1996a), but it was only during the 1990s that its impact became significant, with

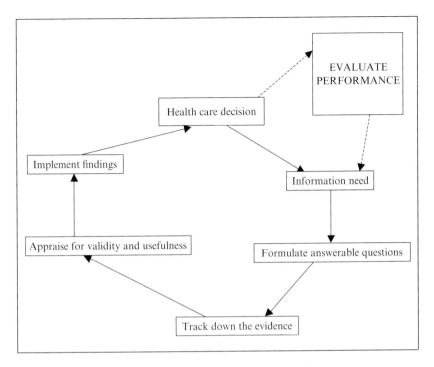

Figure 5.2   Evidence-based decision making within an organisation

libraries and academic centres devoted to its pursuit; courses at undergraduate and postgraduate levels being constructed to meet increasing demand; and training workshops provided across many centres in many countries to spread the message it conveys. Today, EBHC and health technology assessment (HTA) play a significant role in informing decision making at an organisational and health care system level across many countries, with a number of international associations formed to develop research and expertise in the field.

The definition of EBM, which has been widely used, is that provided by Sackett and colleagues: 'Evidence-based medicine is the conscientious, explicit and judicious use of current best evidence in making decisions about the care of individual patients' (Sackett *et al.*, 1996a, p. 71). The authors took great pains to emphasise, however, that 'the practice of EBM means integrating individual clinical expertise with the best available external clinical evidence from systematic research' and that neither *individual clinical expertise* nor *best available external clinical evidence* on its own constituted good clinical practice.

> Without clinical expertise, practice risks becoming tyran-nised by evidence, for even excellent external evidence may be inapplicable to or inappropriate for an individual patient. Without current best evidence, practice risks becoming rapidly out of date, to the detriment of patients.
>
> (Sackett *et al.*, 1996a, p. 71)

However, translating EBM into EBHC requires another dimension – that of patient preferences. Greenhalgh (1996) argues that if it were possible for practice to be completely evidence based a number of theoretical limitations remain, the most important being the complexity of the patient problem and the inability to translate it into a discrete, one-dimensional problem. Furthermore, the most perfect medical remedy, prescribed by a doctor, fully aware of the evidence underlying it, will not translate into an effective treatment if it is not 'owned' by patients, who are prepared to fully comply with the requirements of their treatment regimen. The third feature of EBHC and evidence-based decision making in health care is therefore that of the patient, as reflected in Figure 5.3 below.

The ease with which evidence-based policy making and evidence-based decision making fit into the mould of EBM and EBHC is more contentious. Evidence-based policy mak-ing and evidence-based decision making would appear to have a natural home within a rational model of policy making, as referred to in Chapter 1. The rational policy process cycle described, for example, by Hill (1997) and Nutley & Webb

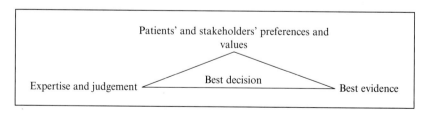

Figure 5.3   Evidence-based decision making

(2000), includes the notion of evaluation and review, and therefore, by implication, research and evidence. We have previously defined evaluation as being 'concerned with judging merit against some yardstick' and involving 'the collection, analysis and interpretation of data . . . attempts to measure the extent to which certain outcomes can be validly correlated with inputs and/or outputs' (Phillips *et al.*, 1994, p. 1), all of which are indicative of the research process and the acquisition of evidence.

However, the criticisms levied at the rational model and the increasing importance attached to incremental models as a feature of pluralistic societies have widened the debate over the role of evidence within the policy making process. For example, Black (2001, p. 275) argues that the 'implicit assumption of a linear relation between research evidence and policy needs to be replaced with a more interactive model'. He highlights a number of reasons why research evidence has little influence on service policies:

- policy makers have goals other than clinical effectiveness, e.g. social, financial, political
- research evidence may be dismissed as irrelevant if generated from a different sector, e.g. the relevance of trials conducted in hospitals for primary care
- lack of consensus about research evidence and its interpretation
- other types of competing evidence, e.g. personal experience, expert opinion
- social environment, e.g. frequent organisational change can dampen morale and hamper introduction of evidence-based approaches
- poor quality of knowledge purveyors, e.g. high turnover rates and lack of expertise among civil servants militate against high quality advice

(Black, 2001, p. 276)

A similar array of constraints hindering the development of evidence-based policy making has been proposed by Leicester (1999) and cited in Nutley & Webb (2000), under the term 'enemies of evidence-based policy'. They highlight seven potential reasons why evidence-based policy is likely to continue to be the exception rather than the rule:

- bureaucratic logic: the logic that says things are right because they have always been done this way
- the bottom line: the logic of the business environment and the throughput measurement that goes with this
- consensus: this involves extensive consultation to find out what matters, followed by an inclusive task force drawn from all interested parties to determine the limits of a solution that will satisfy everyone, which is defined as that which will work
- politics: the art of the possible rather than what is rational or what might work best
- Civil Service culture: in particular a strong distrust of information generated outside the system
- cynicism: an attitude of mind that allows us to go along with the 'company view' or 'conventional wisdom' even though we know it to be false
- time: no wonder there is so little room for evidence-based policy: there is scarcely room even to think

(Nutley & Webb, 2000, p. 36)

However, contrary views are held by Walshe (2001) and Donald (2001), who both argue that the momentum needs to be at least maintained, with the latter arguing that there has been

> a sea change in people's expectation that research should be taken seriously . . . individual doctors, nurses, local managers, health visitors and the public now care enough about research to be palpably frustrated when it cannot be found or implemented . . . taking research seriously – being evidence based – is a discipline requiring decades of work to ensure its support through good times and bad. I do not agree that now is the time to put on the brakes.
>
> (Donald, 2001, p. 279)

It is likely in the short-term future, at least, that there will be greater attempts to bridge the divide between research carried out in academic communities and the use of these findings by politicians and policy makers, with the questions not being restricted to *what works?* but including the questions *when does it work? why does it work? how does it work? under what circumstances does it work?* and summed up under a developed slogan of *Doing the right things right at the right time and under the right conditions.*

The process will inevitably be evolutionary, but it is one which the EBM movement has gone through and which has led policy makers to establish, for example, the Commission for Health Improvement. This body was depicted as an NHS inspectorate by Walshe (1999), but is charged with the overall responsibility for clinical governance and monitoring the quality of care and systems for quality improvement in the UK NHS. In 2004, this body is to be subsumed within the Commission for Healthcare Audit and Inspection, which will aim to:

- accelerate improvement in patient care and health care value for money across England and Wales
- strengthen the accountability for those responsible for the commissioning and delivery of health care
- demonstrate to the public how the additional money being invested in these services is being spent and enable them to judge how performance is improving as a result
- streamline inspection arrangements for healthcare (http://www.doh.gov.uk/statementofpurpose/index.htm)

The locus for these and other policy developments is the notion of clinical governance. This has already been referred to in Chapter 4 but it is also worth considering it briefly here. It was introduced in 1998 as a new approach to the quality improvement in the UK NHS, on the premise that it would be the framework within which health care organisations at every level of the NHS would be 'accountable for monitoring and improving the quality of their services' and it was intended that it would 'safeguard high standards of care by creating an environment in which excellence in clinical care will flourish' (NHS Executive, 1998; Buetow & Roland, 1999). Prior to clinical governance, it had been argued that whereas:

quality assessment and clinical audit were professionally led, quality improvement initiatives involved a shift towards managerial ownership, and quality assurance has been perceived to be either externally driven by managers or to include internal inspection by professionals.

(Buetow & Roland, 1999)

At this time, certain high profile cases of quality lapses, such as paediatric cardiac surgery at Bristol Royal Infirmary and the inability to detect the criminal practices of Harold Shipman and Beverley Allitt, for example, were undermining public confidence in the health care professions and the current bill for clinical negligence stood at £84 million per annum (Fenn *et al.*, 2000). However, a search of the literature to assess whether there was evidence to support the use of clinical governance to improve the quality of patient care concluded that:

as yet, there are no studies providing evidence showing that the adoption of clinical governance brings improvement in the quality of health care, and that these improvements are greater than those of alternative or previously used quality initiatives.

(Thomas, 2001, pp. 253–4)

Other aspects of the policy to establish and deliver quality health care and monitor performance against agreed standards were contained in the formulation of the national service frameworks (NSFs) in priority areas. The intention was that these would be key drivers in modernising the NHS by:

- setting national standards and service models for a defined service or care group
- putting in place strategies to support implementation
- establishing performance milestones against which progress within an agreed timescale will be measured

(http://www.doh.gov.uk/nsf)

In England, at the time of writing, there are NSFs in the areas of mental health, coronary heart disease (CHD), older people and diabetes, with future NSFs planned in renal services, children's services and long-term conditions, focusing on neurological conditions.

The National Institute for Clinical Excellence (NICE) has also formed an important part of the organisational framework for delivering quality improvements and delivering clinically effective services. NICE was set up as a Special Health Authority for England and Wales on 1 April 1999 to provide patients, health professionals and the public with authoritative, robust and reliable guidance on current 'best practice' (http://www.nice.org.uk). The role of NICE has been, to some degree, controversial. Its appraisal of new technologies, an attempt to provide guidance on what constitutes 'best practice' has not been without its detractors (Smith, 2000; Dent & Sadler, 2002; Gafni & Birch, 2003). Its processes involve assessing the clinical evidence relating to medications and therapies, as well as the evidence relating to the cost-effectiveness of such interventions, in order to produce guidance for decision makers within the NHS as to whether such treatments should be made widely available. For example, the key recommendations of the NICE review on treatments for dyspepsia (NICE, 2000) are highlighted in the box below.

Category of dyspepsia	Recommendations
Peptic ulcer	Patients with documented duodenal or gastric ulcers should be tested for *Helicobacter pylori* (HP) and, if positive, should receive eradication therapy – usually a PPI and two antibiotics in high dose for seven days. If they remain symptomatic after eradication, or are HP negative, they should receive a healing dose of PPI, and once healing has been achieved, treatment should be stepped down to the lowest effective dose or stopped.

NSAID-induced ulcers	Patients with documented NSAID-induced ulcers should receive a healing dose of a PPI, followed by a step-down to a maintenance dose which may be given long term.
GORD	Patients with severe GORD should be treated with a healing dose PPI to achieve symptom control followed by a step-down to a maintenance dose. Patients with oesophageal strictures should not be stepped down and should be maintained on healing doses to reduce risk of restricturing. Patients with mild-GORD can be managed on less expensive therapies, using acid suppressants or antacids to control symptoms.
Non-ulcer dyspepsia	Patients with non-ulcer dyspepsia should be treated in a stepped-up or stepped-down approach at the lowest dosage to control symptoms but that they should not be treated with long-term PPIs unless their use is confirmed by endoscopy.

However, it has been claimed that there is ambiguity about how NICE reaches its conclusions and uncertainty about the impact of guidance on the NHS and about who monitors compliance (Dent & Sadler, 2002). Authorities are required to provide appropriate funding for treatments recommended by NICE within three months of the announcement, which may well result in other services being denied funding as a result (Sculpher *et al.*, 2001) and the geographical inequities, which NICE was intended to reduce and remove, being switched to other services.

Managers within the NHS at primary, secondary and tertiary levels, have to be increasingly aware of the need to respond to competing demands on budgets by evidence of the efficacy and cost-effectiveness of various treatments and technologies, which seem to be appearing with increasing frequency. The conflict between endeavouring to meet targets in one area may well run counter to the pressures imposed from another and the evidence-based organisation is one where trade-offs may have to be made. Prior to exploring this in more detail, we need to pay some attention to what actually constitutes *good* evidence?

What constitutes good evidence?

The success of agencies such as NICE and the degree to which other quality initiatives are likely to be embraced are highly dependent on the quality of the information sources which are available, as depicted in Figure 5.2 above. The Cabinet Office (1999), in its attempt to stimulate 'professional policy making' has sought to emphasise the importance of evidence. For example, one of the nine core competences within its model of what an ideal policy making process would look like is to utilise the best evidence from a wide range of sources and involving key stakeholders. It further defines range of sources as expert knowledge, existing domestic and international research, existing statistics, stakeholder consultation, evaluation of previous policies, new research (if appropriate, or secondary sources), including the Internet, costings of policy options and the results of economic or statistical modelling. The document also attempts to broaden the notion of evidence. It states:

> in any policy arena there is a great deal of critical evidence held in the minds of both front-line staff in departments, agencies and local authorities and those to whom the policy is directed.
>
> (Cabinet Office, 1999, paras 7.1 and 7.22)

Table 5.1   Type and strength of evidence (from McQuay & Moore, 1998)

---

(1)   strong evidence from at least one systematic review of multiple well-designed randomised controlled trials

(2)   strong evidence from at least one properly designed randomised controlled trial of appropriate size

(3)   evidence from well-designed trials without randomisation, single group pre-post, cohort, time series or matched case-controlled studies

(4)   evidence from well-designed non-experimental studies from more than one centre or research group

(5)   opinions of respected authorities, based on clinical evidence, descriptive studies or reports of expert committees

---

However, the debate as to what constitutes good evidence reflects the wide range of views relating to the particular paradigm and perspective employed in medical and social science research. Within medicine the positivist approach contrasts strongly with the phenomenological approach, which is more evident in social sciences research. As a consequence, the hierarchy of evidence that exists within EBM, as displayed in Table 5.1, runs counter to the prevailing ethos as to what approaches may be more relevant in the other fields (Macdonald, 2000). Nevertheless, the increase in quality reviews in other fields may help to contribute to 'improve the evidence base and increasing its influence on policy and practice in the public services' (Davies *et al.*, 2000a, p. 361).

The techniques, strengths and limitations of each type of technique for generating evidence have been discussed elsewhere (see, for example, Gray, 1997) and will not be further explored here. Rather, the issue is whether the evidence can fulfil three basic requirements:

● are the results valid: can they be believed; have the studies conformed to recognised practice and procedures; to what extent have bias and other external factors impacted on the research; which outcomes were considered and are they meaningful?

- what are the results: does the intervention work as intended; what are the risks that the intervention will cause harm; how precise are they; is there wide variation across the findings?
- how relevant are the results: can they apply in different environments and different settings?

However, within the evidence-based organisation, there are many other decisions that do not fall within these parameters, for example, decisions relating to staff development, staff appraisal and staff selection. Furthermore, as we have noted in Chapters 3 and 4, policy making and decision making within organisations tend to be complex, diverse and context and culture dependent. In the field of public health, for example, it has been argued that the criteria used to assess evidence within clinical practice may not be sufficiently extensive to:

> distinguish between the fidelity of the evaluation process in detecting the success or failure of an intervention, and the success or failure of the intervention itself. Moreover, if an intervention is unsuccessful, the evidence should help to determine whether the intervention was inherently faulty (that is, failure of intervention concept or theory), or just badly delivered (failure of implementation).
>
> (Rychetnik *et al.*, 2002, p. 119)

They further argue that:

> proper interpretation of the evidence depends upon the availability of descriptive information on the intervention and its context, so that the transferability of the evidence can be determined. Study design alone is an inadequate marker of evidence quality in public health intervention evaluation.
>
> (Rychetnik *et al.*, 2002, p. 126)

In summary, therefore, what constitutes best evidence within the context of the evidence-based organisation must take account of the circumstances and conditions prevailing within the organisation and its environment. In addition, the three requirements highlighted above need to be supplemented by other relevant considerations:

- what are the implications of applying these findings within the current organisational dynamics?
- to what extent would the implications of findings cause destabilisation within the organisation?
- would there need to be significant change if these findings were to be implemented?
- what would be the reaction of service users and other stakeholders to the findings?
- what are the resource implications resulting from implementing such evidence?
- are there alternative perspectives that need to be considered?

Reporting evidence

Within an evidence-based organisation the time required to engage fully in the evidence-based decision making process is likely to be inversely proportional to the actual time available to search, analyse and digest such information. Fortunately, 'short-cuts' are available, which have developed as information technology has both opened up and speeded up information transfer. The availability of online electronic journals and databases, alongside publications that are specifically designed to synthesise and disseminate information relating to the effectiveness of interventions, has provided a basis for improved decision making. However, the old adage still holds that the quality of decision making is directly proportional to the information that informs such decisions. It has been argued that 'systematic reviews of inadequate quality may be worse than none, because faulty decisions may be made with unjustified confidence' (McQuay & Moore, 1998, p. 32). Therefore, quality checks need to be in place at all stages of the *evidence-based process*, from the initial search strategy to the final reporting of information.

There are many sources of criteria for assessing the quality of research (see for example, Sackett *et al.*, 1991; Schultz *et al.*, 1995; Jadad *et al.*, 1996; Gray, 1997; Greenhalgh, 1997; McQuay & Moore, 1998; Moore *et al.*, 2003). For example, Moore *et al.* (2003) report on the Oxford quality scoring system, where points are awarded according to whether the trial was randomised, whether it was double-blinded, and whether any withdrawals were described. A five-rated randomised controlled trial would, therefore, have its randomisation process clearly stated, using appropriate procedures; it would be performed by investigators who were blinded to which patient received intervention and placebo; the patients would also be blind as to who received intervention and placebo; and patient withdrawals would be documented and reported.

Similarly, considerable energy and effort has been used in EBM to develop ways of reporting evidence, with many sources now available for the interested reader (for example, Donald & Haines, 1998; Haines & Silagy, 1998; Greenhalgh & Donald, 2000; Sackett *et al.*, 2000; Tramèr, 2000; Moore *et al.*, 2003) and the following web-pages:

- http://www.jr2.ox.ac.uk/bandolier/painres/download/whatis/whatis.html
- http://www.jr2.ox.ac.uk/bandolier/booth/booths/ebmstor.html
- http://cebm.jr2.ox.ac.uk/
- http://www.med.ualberta.ca/ebm/ebm.htm
- http://www.ebmny.org/
- http://www.cochrane.org/

The developments within the EBM field have brought with them 'ready-made quality checked information' and led to claims that 'we should burn our (traditional) textbooks and trade in our (traditional) journal subscriptions because there are now better resources for keeping current' (Sackett *et al.*, 2000, p. 34). In terms of evidence-based decision making and policy making, the field is not as developed and much more work needs to be undertaken in determining what constitutes good evidence and how it can be accessed. However, there is an increasing need to ensure that health care managers move to a position where they avoid implementing policies that do not work and ensure that they implement policies that work.

Too often and for too long the evaluation of policies has been viewed as a 'necessary add-on' rather than an important factor in determining whether the policy should or should not be implemented in the first place.

Presentation of evidence

As well as facilitating ease of access to evidence it is also important that decision makers receive available quality evidence in bite-size chunks. It is highly debatable whether many decision makers ever venture into the inner depths of reports beyond the 'executive summary' and whether they would entangle themselves with the details and intricacies contained in many scientific papers let alone systematic reviews. If evidence is to affect practice it must reach the recipients(s) it is intended to influence. Proponents of EBM have spent many hours and pages to facilitate ease of access to quality evidence, which can influence practice and improve patient care.

However, a simple linear relationship between evidence/ knowledge and receipt oversimplifies the generalisability of research evidence according to Nutley & Davies (2000). They refer to the need for 'reflective transfer' (Schon, 1987), which basically refers to the assessment of the research findings to the situation and circumstances, and a recognition of the importance of tacit knowledge or 'craft knowledge' (Hargreaves, 1999), which is inherent in being a professional (Schon, 1991). The picture of evidence-based decision making portrayed in Figure 5.2, indicates that expertise and knowledge also need to encompass this tacit knowledge. Other factors, highlighted by Nutley & Davies (2000) under the umbrella of broad influences on practice, also need to be brought on board. The six broad categories they identify are:

- research evidence and declarative knowledge
- organisational resources
- organisational structures and cultural norms
- service user demands and pressure from other stakeholders

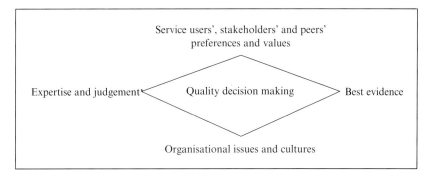

Figure 5.4 Evidence-based decision making in public service organisations

- peer values and pressures
- routines and craft/procedural knowledge
   (Nutley & Davies, 2000, pp. 337–8)

These factors, although not necessarily exhaustive, are particularly relevant for evidence-based decision making and evidence-based policy making, and lead to a restatement of the triangle in Figure 5.3 to embrace inter-organisational and intra-organisational issues and cultures, as shown in Figure 5.4.

However, it is also worth emphasising that the transaction costs associated with moving towards evidence-based decision making and joined-up thinking in both decision making and policy making are not insubstantial. The ability, therefore, to develop and utilise presentational techniques, which provide meaningful and comprehensible information effectively and efficiently for managers to synthesise and appraise within the overall perspective of the evidence-based organisation (Gray, 1997) is one of the aspects of EBM that should be warmly welcomed. The EBM movement has invested considerable energies into the most effective ways of disseminating and presenting good quality information and interested readers are invited to access some of the potential sources (for example, Laupacis *et al.*, 1994; Cook & Sackett, 1995; Sackett, 1996; Sackett *et al.*, 1996b; McQuay and Moore, 1997).

Application of evidence

The emphasis on evidence and quality in policy documenta-
tion will only bear fruit in practice if relevant research findings
and valid guideline recommendations become part of normal
practice and organisational environments are adjusted to
facilitate such approaches. We have already highlighted the
potential constraints that organisational cultures can have
on translating evidence into practice. The multifaceted complexities of organisational cultures and politics are compounded by the variability in personalities of which they are
composed, all of which combine to produce a spectrum of
outcomes which may range from explosive failures to highly
successful programmes and policies. More work needs to be
done to assess the effectiveness of intra-organisational, inter-
organisational, inter-professional, collaborative and partnership approaches to the organisation and delivery of services
in order to accompany the wealth of research evidence relating to practice (El Ansari *et al.*, 2001; El Ansari & Phillips,
2001).

There are also other costs associated with the application
of evidence, which need to be mentioned. The large number
of journals delivered to every practitioner and manager in
the course of a week and the volume of material available on
the Web adds to the already severe pressures on them to
read, appraise and determine its relevance to their particular
situations. This obviously presupposes that the desire to adopt
and utilise evidence-based information is present. However,
it has been demonstrated that 'the naive assumption that
when research information is made available it is some-
how accessed by practitioners, appraised and then applied
in practice is now largely discredited' (NHS CRD, 1999).
Indeed, it has been argued (Weiss, 1998) that much research
appears to have very little or no impact on practice. Weiss
further argues that to think about the use of research evidence without considering the organisational context is to
miss a large part of the story. The EBO, she argues, needs to
remove impediments to new ways of working and more often

to supply supportive structures, which incorporate and sustain new initiatives and activities.

Evidence relating to the effectiveness of interventions aimed at achieving changing practice has been documented by the Effective Practice and Organisation of Care (EPOC) Review Group within the Cochrane Collaboration (NHS CRD, 1999). What they have argued is that multifaceted interventions (which combine two or more of: audit and feedback, reminders, local consensus processes and marketing) seem to be more effective than single interventions. For example, research has shown that well constructed educational programmes (educational outreach) that take the message to professionals can be reasonably successful.

Pawson & Tilley (1997) argued that the complexities and potential conflicts which exist within organisations at any one point in time make it compulsory to know not only *what* works but also *why*, and in *what circumstances*, it works and does not work. As we noted in Chapter 4, the foundations on which these issues are based are explored by Nutley & Davies (2000), who conclude that, 'there is much to be gained from viewing evidence-influenced practice as a partnership activity' (p. 342). They advocate an approach that combines:

- insights from systems thinking (in terms of setting the contexts within which evidence is to be used)
- understanding of individual decision making and behaviour change (which acknowledges the importance of craft routines and tacit knowledge by professionals)
- awareness that the nature of the innovation being promulgated will influence its diffusion (and in particular, the 'fit' between the innovation, the context and those who are potential adopters)
- ownership of evidence through partnerships in the evidence generation process.

(Nutley & Davies, 2000, pp. 342–3)

In summary, the ratio of cost/benefit in applying evidence is crucial in determining the speed at which the evidence-based organisation develops. If the costs of changing behaviour are greater than the benefits resulting from change then it may be preferable to retain the status quo. Because of the workings of health care systems, new, important, and cost effective treatments sometimes do not become routine care, while well marketed products of equivocal value achieve widespread adoption. The question has been asked whether managers should attempt to influence clinical behaviour and adjust for these inefficient practices, while the conclusion reached is that trying to improve the uptake of underused cost-effective care or reduce the overuse of new and expensive treatments may not always make economic sense (Mason *et al.*, 2001).

Outcomes

> The ward was full, so I put him in my room as he was moribund and screaming and I did not want to take him to the ward. I examined him. He had obvious gross bilateral cavitation and a severe pleural rub. I thought the latter was the cause of the pain and screaming. I had no morphia, just aspirin, which had no effect. I felt desperate. I knew very little Russian then and there was no one in the ward who did. I finally instinctively sat down on the bed and took him in my arms, and the screaming stopped almost at once. He died peacefully in my arms a few hours later. It was not the pleurisy that caused the screaming, but loneliness. It was a wonderful education about the care of the dying. I was ashamed of my misdiagnosis and kept the story secret.
>
> (in Cochrane & Blythe, 1989)

This is an account of one episode during Archie Cochrane's years spent in prisoner of war camps in Salonika and Germany. It illustrates many points, but one which is particularly relevant here. Cochrane's original diagnosis of cause and effect may well have been clinically accurate but even in the presence of appropriate medication, would not have secured an appropriate outcome from the patient's perspective. This was only achieved when Cochrane resorted to his instincts, brought about as a result of desperation in the situation. It serves to illustrate that in any given situation there are a multiplicity of possible outcomes, the significance of which is dependent on the perspective being considered – that of the patient, the professional, the manager, the funding agency, or any other stakeholder.

For example, what should be regarded as outcome measures in health promotion or palliative care? In the former, many studies have relied on mortality reduction, or variations on this theme – for example, avoidable life years lost (Godfrey *et al.*, 1989) – as an indicator of effectiveness. However, this is not very appropriate where interventions have a greater impact on morbidity or aspects relating to quality of life. Whereas well-years and QALYs would enable the combination of mortality and morbidity factors, there is also a case for distinguishing between the implications for mortality and the impact on morbidity from changes in behaviour relating to 'health-damaging' activities (Nutbeam *et al.*, 1991). But, in addition, the nature of health promotion activities necessitates the use of process indicators and intermediate outcomes (Tolley, 1993; Whelan *et al.*, 1993) or indirect, intermediate, behavioural, subjective and clinical indicators (Tones, 1992; Tones & Tilford, 1994). These more subjective indicators highlight the need for evaluations to utilise appropriate outcome measures, which fully take into account the nature and scope of the programme and its alternatives.

In addition, the recognition of the importance of the patient's perspective in the monitoring and evaluation of health care has brought with it numerous approaches to the measurement of what has been termed 'subjective well being' (Jenkinson & McGee, 2002), the aim of which is to provide more accurate assessment of individuals' or populations' health and the benefits and harms that may result from interventions (Fitzpatrick *et al.*, 1992). This is particularly evident when considering the objective of care provided by the hospice movement – to give patients an opportunity to live to their fullest in physical ease and the assurance of personal relationships until death, rather than having the curing function as the major focus (Saunders & Baines, 1989). The hospice movement had, in fact, grown out of a sense of dissatisfaction with the prevailing systems of health care that were relatively poor in providing effective pain relief and symptom control and which ignored the emotional, social and spiritual needs of the dying person (Clark, 1993). The movement has attempted to demonstrate that a deterioration in the quality of life is neither an inevitable nor a necessary consequence of becoming terminally ill (Field & James, 1993) and in so doing, has restored the caring art of medicine in its approach to the tending of the dying and their families (Dunlop & Hockley, 1990).

Gray (1997) develops the issues relating to outcomes further by arguing that once it has been demonstrated that the research is of sufficient quality for the outcomes to be considered relevant for the decision making process, the outcomes must be assessed using five key questions:

- how many outcomes were studied?
- how large were the effects found?
- with what degree of confidence can the results be applied to the whole population?
- does the intervention do more good than harm?
- how relevant are the results to the 'local' population or service about which the decision is being made?

(Gray, 1997, p. 103)

Outcomes may not always be positive and both benefit and harm need to be considered, since few treatments benefit every patient (Gray, 1997). We noted in Chapter 4 that, for example, NSAIDs are highly effective analgesics, provide protection against cardiovascular events and have other potential benefits, but also lead to a threefold to ten-fold increase in ulcer complications, hospitalisation and death (Seager & Hawkey, 2001). Moore & Phillips (1999) estimated that the number of patients admitted to hospital with upper gastrointestinal crises, resulting from NSAID use, for an average primary care group (PGC) of 100 000 patients was 24 per year. For the average GP, with a list size of less than one tenth of the PGC, the number would be around 2 patients per year and probably no great significance would have been given to such outcomes. However, the impact at PGC level is much more noticeable and significant in terms of overall budgets, and calls for an analysis of prescribing strategies and a move towards what may be termed *joined-up decision making*.

However, many of the problems result from decision making being fragmented and narrowly focused, with excessive significance attached to financial budgets, with drug costs often targeted for cutbacks, since they are easy to measure, while other major costs and sources of waste are ignored (Smith, 2001). However, it has been argued that the cost of treatment is not simply the cost of drugs or medical and nursing time but includes recovery times, incidence of side effects, rate of delayed discharge, use of care resources post-discharge (community and primary care, social services and costs to patients and their families) and the cost of system deficiencies and problems (Phillips, 2003).

In this context, we believe the move to unified, cash limited budgets within primary care is a move in the right direction. GPs will have to take more responsibility for determining priorities and controlling prescribing and hospital budgets, which should act as a stimulus to develop cost-effective prescribing. For example, prescribing decisions intended to ensure that drug budgets were not exceeded, now need to be made within a wider context, since the administration of a relatively high cost drug may well prevent even more expensive hospital admissions, thereby producing a net benefit in terms of the overall budget and patient outcomes. The Audit Commission (2001) implicitly advocated this joined-up approach to decision making rather than one driven by a narrow budgetary focus:

> In recent years, these cost pressures have been driven by the introduction of new medicines. . . . These cost pressures are cause for concern for many trust boards, but they need to be viewed as part of the overall package of patient care. For some conditions, medicines expenditure should be rising because it would be a cost-effective way of increasing the health gain for the population. For example,

expenditure on proton pump inhibitors and H2 antagonists should be rising because their use improves the quality of patients' lives and saves money by preventing invasive surgery.

(Audit Commission, 2001)

Decisions relating to which services and treatments should be provided are highly complex and involve a number of different, often conflicting, factors. Economic evaluation techniques are often used by decision makers to utilise information relating to the effectiveness, the efficiency and equity of interventions and programmes in order to enhance the quality of the commissioning process in determining health care priorities and in ensuring that the best care is provided within available resources.

The integration of evidence relating to effectiveness and resource utilisation can be brought together in a matrix (Donaldson & Mugford, 2002) as shown in Figure 5.5 below, or with threshold values attached. For example, interventions with cost-QALY ratios of between £3 000 and £20 000 were adjudged to be cost-effective when there was good clinical evidence of their effectiveness (Stevens *et al.*, 1995), while it has been argued that NICE is more likely to view a technology favourably, subject to other relevant factors, if it costs less that £30 000 per QALY (Towse & Pritchard, 2003).

Joined-up thinking and decision making within the health service itself needs to be part of joined-up policy making on the part of Government. A successful outcome in one policy arena can have highly significant negative outcomes in another. For example, after the Hatfield railway crash in October 2000 *The Economist* argued that 'Britain spends too much money, not too little, making its railways safe' (*The Economist*, 2000a) and 'that overreaction to last month's rail crash has increased the risks to rail passengers, not reduced them' by making it more difficult to travel by rail resulting in people increasing their reliance on car travel – which is much more risky than rail travel (*The Economist*, 2000b). It concluded that:

Declining effectiveness

		1	2	3	4
Increasing cost	A	y	y	j	n
	B	y	y/n	n	n
	C	j	n	n	n
	D	n	n	n	n

y = yes adopt
n = no reject
y/n = indifferent
j = judgement needed

EFFECTIVENESS
Compared with control the intervention has:
1 evidence of greater effectiveness
2 evidence of no difference in effectiveness
3 evidence of less effectiveness
4 not enough evidence of effectiveness

COST
Compared with control the intervention has:
A evidence of cost savings
B evidence of no difference in costs
C evidence of greater costs
D not enough evidence on costs

Figure 5.5 Integration of effectiveness and resource utilisation evidence (based on Donaldson, Mugford & Vale, 2002)

From society's point of view it is far from rational to spend 150 times as much on saving a life on the railways as on saving a life on the roads. A bereaved mother cares little how her child was killed. Many more lives could be saved if the money currently being poured into avoiding spectacular but rare railway crashes were spent instead on avoiding the tragedies that happen ten times every day on the roads.

(*The Economist*, 2000a)

When evaluating the effectiveness of its policy on railway safety against the model of professional policy making produced by the Cabinet Office (1999) it is clear that it does not meet many of the competences identified earlier as encapsulating the key elements of the policy making process. It is clear that political expediency remains a major driver in policy making, while many philosophical and ethical issues remain to be discussed before we can say that the evidence-based organisation has truly arrived. The need for further attention to these issues has been advocated by one of the originators of the concepts of EBM (Haynes, 2002) and it is these matters that the next chapter addresses.

Summary

What we have tried to demonstrate here, against the context of the model displayed in Chapter 1, on page 4, is that against a background of limited resources trying to satisfy infinite wants, needs, desires and demands, the need for high quality evidence to be made accessible for managerial decision making is essential. The rational model, which is heavily reliant on information and evaluation to drive the policy process, is therefore dependent on decisions that are driven by evidence rather than whim or inappropriate power. However, the actual process of decision making and indeed policy making requires that evidence itself forms only one of the constituent parts that make up the process of good quality decision making. The ability to relate evidence and assess its suitability and applicability to the organisational context and culture is another feature of the evidence-based organisation, and one which requires considerable skill and expertise on the part of decision makers and policy makers.

In Chapter 3, we drew attention to the multiple rationalities that managers in health care systems are obliged to acknowledge. In this chapter, the need for more rational, cost effective decision making has been advocated through the various sources of evidence relating to clinical interventions. The evidence-based organisation is expected to consider the economic and socio-cultural contexts in which it seeks to respond to the populations' health needs. Yet the context itself is largely determined by the priorities for spending in certain health areas, such as cancer, cardiovascular disease and mental health, which have been decided at a macro-political level. Managers, therefore, have to operate in the real world of politics, where short-term expediency tends to relegate rational approaches, even based on the best available evidence, to the list of considered but sometimes rejected options.

References

Audit Commission (2001) *A spoonful of sugar: medicines management in NHS hospitals*. Audit Commission, London.

Black, N. (2001) 'Evidence-based policy: proceed with care'. *British Medical Journal*, **323**, 275–8.

Borowitz, M. & Sheldon, T. (1993) 'Controlling health care: from economic interventions to micro-clinical regulation'. *Health Economics*, **2**, 201–204.

Buetow, S.A. & Roland, M. (1999) 'Clinical governance: bridging the gap between managerial and clinical approaches to quality of care'. *Quality in Health Care*, **8** (3), 184–90.

Cabinet Office – Strategic policy Making Team (1999) *Professional policy making for the twentyfirst century*. Cabinet Office, London.

Clark, D. (1993) 'Whither the hospices?' In: *The Future for Palliative Care* (ed. Clark, D.). Open University Press, Buckingham.

Cochrane, A.L. & Blythe, M. (1989) *One man's medicine: an autobiography of Professor Archie Cochrane*. British Medical Journal Memoir Club, London.

Cook, R.J. & Sackett, D.L. (1995) 'The number needed to treat: a clinically useful measure of treatment effect'. *British Medical Journal*, **310**, 452–4.

Davies, H.T.O., Nutley, S.M. & Mannion, R. (2000b) 'Organisational culture and quality of health care'. *Quality in Health Care*, **9**, 11–19.

Davies, H.T.O., Nutley, S.M. & Smith, P.C. (2000a) 'Learning from the past, prospects for the future'. In: *What works? Evidence-based policy and practice in public services* (eds Davies, H.T.O., Nutley, S.M. & Smith, P.C.). The Policy Press, Bristol.

Dent, T.H.S. & Sadler, M. (2002) 'From guidance to practice: why NICE is not enough'. *British Medical Journal*, **324**, 842–5.

Donald, A. (2001) 'Research must be taken seriously'. *British Medical Journal*, **323**, 278–9.

Donald, A. & Greenhalgh, T. (1999) *A hands-on guide to evidence-based health care: practice and implementation.* Blackwell, Oxford.

Donald, A. & Haines, A. (1998) *Getting Research Findings into Practice.* BMJ Books, London.

Donaldson, C., Mugford, M. & Vale, L. (2002) 'Using systematic reviews in economic evaluation: the basic principles'. In: *Evidence-based health economics: from effectiveness to efficiency in systematic review* (eds Donaldson, C., Mugford, M. & Vale, L.). BMJ Books, London.

Dunlop, R.J. & Hockley, J.M. (1990) *Terminal care support teams, the hospital-hospice interface.* Oxford University Press, Oxford.

El Ansari, W., Phillips, C.J. & Hammick, M. (2001) 'Collaboration and partnerships: developing the evidence base'. *Health and Social Care in the Community*, **9** (4), 215–27.

El Ansari, W. & Phillips, C.J. (2001) 'Interprofessional collaboration: a stakeholder approach to evaluation of voluntary participation in community partnerships'. *Journal of Interprofessional Care*, **15** (4), 351–68.

Fenn, P., Diacon, S., Gray, A., Hodges, R. & Rickman, N. (2000) 'Current cost of medical negligence in NHS hospitals: analysis of claims database'. *British Medical Journal*, June 10, **320** (7249), 1567–71.

Field, D. & James, J. (1993) 'Where and how people die'. In: *The Future for Palliative Care* (ed. Clark, D.). Open University Press, Buckingham.

Fitzpatrick, R., Fletcher, A., Gore, S., Jones, D., Spiegelhalter, D. & Cox, D. (1992) 'Quality of life measures in health care. I: applications and issues in assessment'. *British Medical Journal*, **305**, 1074–7.

Gafni, A. & Birch, S. (2003) 'NICE methodological guidelines and decision making in the National Health Service in England and Wales'. *Pharmacoeconomics*, **21** (3), 149–57.

Godfrey, C., Hardman, G. & Maynard, A. (1989) 'Priorities for health promotion: an economic approach'. Discussion Paper 59, Centre for Health Economics, University of York, York.

Gray, J.A.M. (1997) Evidence-based health care: how to make health policy and management decisions. Churchill Livingstone, Edinburgh.

Greenhalgh, T. (1996) 'Is my practice evidence based?' *British Medical Journal*, **313**, 957–8.

Greenhalgh, T. (1997) *How to read a paper: the basics of evidence based medicine.* BMJ Books, London.

Greenhalgh, T. & Donald, A. (2000) *Evidence Based Health Care Workbook.* BMJ Books, London.

Haines, A. & Silagy, C. (1998) *Evidence Based Practice in Primary Health Care.* BMJ Books, London.

Hargreaves, D. (1999) 'Can and should evidence inform policy and practice in education?' Evidence-based practices and policies seminar, 22 June 1999. The Royal Society, London.

Haynes, R.B. (2002) 'What kind of evidence is it that evidence-based medicine advocates want health care providers and consumers to pay attention to?' BMC Health Services Research, **2**, 3. Biothed Central (http://www.biomedcentral.com/172–6963/2/3).

Hill, M. (1997) 'The policy process in the modern state'. Prentice Hall and Wheatsheaf, London.

Jadad, A.R., Moore, R.A., Carroll, D., Jenkinson, C., Reynolds, D.J., Gavaghan, D.J. & McQuay, H.J. (1996) 'Assessing the quality of reports of randomised clinical trials: is blinding necessary?' *Controlled Clinical Trials*, **17**, 1–12.

Jenkinson, C. & McGee, H. (2002) 'Patient assessed outcomes: measuring health status and quality of life'. In: *Assessment and evaluation of health and medical care* (ed. Jenkinson, C.). Open University Press, Buckingham.

Laupacis, A., Sackett, D.L. & Roberts, R.S. (1994) 'An assessment of clinically useful measures of the consequences of treatment'. *New England Journal of Medicine*, **318**, 1728–33.

Leicester, G. (1999) 'The seven enemies of evidence-based policy'. *Public Money and Management*, **19**, 5–7.

Macdonald, G. (2000) 'Social care: rhetoric and reality'. In: *What works? Evidence-based policy and practice in public services* (eds Davies, H.T.O., Nutley, S.M. & Smith, P.C.). The Policy Press, Bristol.

Mason, J., Freemantle, N., Nazareth, I., Eccles, M., Haines, A. & Drummond, M. (2001) When is it cost-effective to change the behavior of health professionals? *Journal of the American Medical Association*, **286**, 2988–92.

McQuay, H.J. & Moore, R.A. (1997) 'Using numerical results from systematic reviews in clinical practice'. *Annals of Internal Medicine*, **126**, 712–20.

McQuay, H.J. & Moore, R.A. (1998) *An evidence-based resource for pain relief*. Oxford University Press, Oxford.

Moore, R.A., Edwards, J., Barden, J. & McQuay, H.J. (2003) *Bandolier's Little Book of Pain: an evidence-based guide to treatments*. Oxford University Press, Oxford.

Moore, R.A. & Phillips, C.J. (1999) Cost of NSAID adverse effects to the UK National Health Service. *Journal of Medical Economics*, **2**, 45–55.

NHS Executive (1998) *A first class service*. Department of Health, London.

National Institute of Clinical Excellence (2000) *The appropriate use of proton pump inhibitors in the treatment of dyspepsia*. National Institute of Clinical Excellence Technology Appraisal Guidance, No. 7. NICE, London.

National Institute of Clinical Excellence (2001) *Guidance on the use of cyclo-oxygenase (Cox) II selective inhibitors, celecoxib, rofecoxib, meloxicam and etodolac for osteoarthritis and rheumatoid arthritis*. National Institute of Clinical Excellence Technology Appraisal Guidance, No. 27. NICE, London.

NHS Centre for Reviews and Disssemination (1999) 'Getting research into practice'. *Effective Health Care Bulletin*, **5**, 1. Royal Society of Medicine Press, London.

Nutbeam, D., Prowle, M. & Phillips, C.J. (1991) 'The Heartbeat Wales No-smoking Intervention: an empirical study of the economic viability of a health promotion programme'. *Heartbeat Wales*, Technical Report 22. Health Promotion Authority for Wales, Cardiff.

Nutley, S.M. & Davies, H.T.O. (2000) 'Making a reality of evidence-based practice'. In: *What works? Evidence-based policy and practice in public services* (eds Davies, H.T.O., Nutley, S.M. & Smith, P.C.). The Policy Press, Bristol.

Nutley, S.M. & Webb, J. (2000) 'Evidence and the policy process'. In: *What works? Evidence-based policy and practice in public services* (eds Davies, H.T.O., Nutley, S.M. & Smith, P.C.). The Policy Press, Bristol.

Pawson, R. & Tilley, N. (1997) *Realistic Evaluation*. Sage, London.

Phillips, C.J. (1997) *Economic evaluation and health promotion*. Avebury, Aldershot.

Phillips, C.J. (2003) 'Cost effectiveness of anaesthesia and analgesia'. In: *Evidence based resource in anaesthesia and analgesia* (ed. Tramér, M.). BMJ Books, London.

Phillips, C.J., Palfrey, C.F. & Thomas, P. (1994) *Evaluating health and social care*. Macmillan, London.

Phillips, C.J. & Prowle, M.J. (1992) 'Evaluating a health campaign: the Heartbeat Wales no-smoking initiative'. *Contemporary Wales*, **5**, 187–212.

Rychetnik, L., Frommer, M., Hawe, P. & Shiell, A. (2002) 'Criteria for evaluating evidence on public health interventions'. *Journal of Epidemiology and Community Health*, **56**, 119–27.

Sackett, D.L. (1996) 'On some clinically useful measures on the effects of treatment'. *Evidence-Based Medicine*, **1**, 37–8.

Sackett, D.L., Deeks, J.J. & Altman, D.G. (1996b) 'Down with odds ratios!'. *Evidence Based Medicine*, **1**, 164–6.

Sackett, D.L., Haynes, R.B., Guyatt, G.H. & Tugwell, P. (1991) *Clinical epidemiology: a basic science for clinical medicine*. Little Brown, London.

Sackett, D.L., Rosenberg, W.M.C., Gray, J.A.M., Haynes, R.B. & Richardson, W.S. (1996a) 'Evidence based medicine: what it is and what it isn't'. *British Medical Journal*, **312**, 71.

Sackett, D.L., Straus, S., Richardson, W.S., Rosenburg, W.M.C. & Haynes, R.B. (2000) *Evidence-based Medicine: How to practice and teach EBM*. Churchill Livingstone, London.

Saunders, C. & Baines, M. (1989) *Living with dying: the management of terminal disease*. Oxford Medical Publications, Oxford.

Schon, D.A. (1987) *Educating the reflective practitioner: toward a new design for teaching and learning in the professions.* Jossey-Bass, San Francisco, Calif.

Schon, D.A. (1991) *The reflective practitioner.* Ashgate Publishing, Aldershot.

Schultz, K.F., Chalmers, I., Hayes, R.J. & Altman, D.G. (1995) 'Empirical evidence of bias: dimensions of methodological quality associated with estimates of treatment effects in controlled trials'. *Journal of the American Medical Association,* **273**, 408–12.

Sculpher, M., Drummond, M. & O'Brien, B. (2001) 'Effectiveness, efficiency and NICE'. *British Medical Journal,* **322**, 943–4.

Seager, J.M. & Hawkey, C.J. (2001) 'Indigestion and non-steroidal anti-inflammatory drugs'. *British Medical Journal,* **323**, 1236–9.

Smith, I. (2001) 'Cost considerations in the use of anaesthetic drugs'. *Pharmacoeconomics,* **19**, 469–81.

Smith, R. (2000) 'The failings of NICE'. *British Medical Journal,* **321**, 1363–4.

Stevens, A., Colin-Jones, D. & Gabbay, J. (1995) 'Quick and Clean: authoritative health technology assessment for local health care contracting'. *Health Trends,* **27**, 37–42.

The Economist (2000a) 'The price of safety'. *The Economist,* 23 November.

The Economist (2000b) 'How not to run a railway'. *The Economist,* 23 November.

Thomas, M. (2001) 'The evidence base for clinical governance'. *Journal of Evaluation in Clinical Practice,* **8**, 251–4.

Tolley, K. (1993) *Health promotion: how to measure cost-effectiveness.* Health Promotion Authority, London.

Tones, B.K. (1992) 'Measuring success in health promotion: selecting indicators of performance'. *Hygie,* **11**, 10–14.

Tones, B.K. & Tilford, S. (1994) *Health Education: effectiveness, efficiency and equity.* Chapman Hall, London.

Towse, A. & Pritchard, C. (2003) 'Does NICE have a threshold? An external view'. In: *Cost-effectiveness thresholds: economic and ethical issues* (eds Towse, A., Pritchard, C. & Devlin, N.). Office of Health Economics, London.

Tramèr, M. (2000) *An Evidence-Based Resource in Anaesthesia and Analgesia.* BMJ Books, London.

Walshe, K. (1999) 'Improvement through inspection? The development of the new Commission for Health Improvement in England and Wales'. *Quality in Health Care,* **8**, 191–6.

Walshe, K. (2001) 'Evidence based policy: don't be timid'. *British Medical Journal,* **323**, 187.

Warner, M. & Evans, W. (1993) 'Pearls of wisdom'. *Health Service Journal,* 16 September.

Whelan, A., Murphy, S. & Smith, C. (1993) 'Performance indicators in health promotion: a review of possibilities and problems'. *Health Promotion Wales*, Technical Report 2. Health Promotion Wales, Cardiff.

Weiss, C.H. (1998) 'Have we learned anything new about the use of evaluation?' *American Journal of Evaluation*, **19**, 21–33.

Chapter 6
Politics, Ethics and
Health Care Management

There are four major dimensions to policy making at government level (Palfrey, 2000). They are *political*, *ideological*, *financial* and *moral*. At any one time, all or some of these concerns will be implicit or explicit in the process of selecting from options. In a very real sense, as we have argued elsewhere, evaluation is inherently a political process (Palfrey & Thomas, 1999). Those elected to power have an obvious wish to retain that power. Therefore, decisions regarding which issues to consider as part of the political agenda and which to discard – described by Hogwood & Gunn (1984) as 'issue filtration' – will be strongly influenced by pragmatic views of potential electoral benefits or disadvantages.

But, from time to time, a government will pursue a policy that ostensibly is unpopular among the electorate. The decision to engage in a war against Iraq in 2003 is a notable example of a Prime Minister appearing to implement a decision that was opposed by a majority of the public and by a significant number of MPs in his own Government. Decisions of this nature – a previous Conservative Prime Minister's refusal to retract the reform of local taxation (the 'poll tax') is another example – are usually regarded by political commentators as personally and collectively hazardous for those making the decisions. Time will tell whether Mr Blair's decision will have adverse consequences in terms of electoral or personal repercussions. We know that the poll tax spelled the beginning of the end of Mrs Thatcher's political career and that her original intention to introduce swingeing changes in the NHS had to be tempered in the light of prospective electoral fallout (Baggott, 1998).

At organisational level, as we shall indicate later in this chapter, pragmatic considerations will feature prominently in managerial decisions or recommendations. At both Government and organisation levels, crucial questions about which services should receive which share of the budget have to be resolved. NHS trusts and primary care organisations, as well as strategic health authorities in England and regional offices in Wales, must have regard to priorities and targets set by the Government of the day. Political decisions, therefore, reduce the autonomy of managers and medical practitioners to executive and administrative levels of jurisdiction in various areas of decision making.

The dictum from Lee & Mills (1985), that policy making is concerned both with what is politically feasible and technically desirable, neatly encapsulates the importance for health care managers of balancing *what should be done* with *what can be done* – a recognition of the *realpolitik* of the management position. Furthermore, successful managers are likely to be blessed with sensitive antennae that can pick up what Veney & Kaluzny (1984) called 'unstated agendas'. For example, the move towards the community as the preferred location for a variety of previously hospital based services was presented in official policy statements as a recognition of people's rights to remain in their own homes wherever possible. Domiciliary health and social care services were to be organised in a seamless form of provision as a response to a kind of moral imperative. This was the emphasis in the White Paper of 1989 which followed the *Griffiths Report* of the previous year.

We know, however, that the Audit Commission's report of 1986 had focused exclusively on the mounting demands on Government budgets from heavily subsidised residential care. For people who could not afford private care, the costs were met from the benefits system, a recourse depicted by the report as a 'perverse incentive'. The policy to divert provision from hospital and residential locations to 'the community' was primarily financial although this preoccupation was partly submerged beneath the explicitly humane argument of individuals' rights.

This critique is not intended to offer a cynical interpretation of policy presentation. Governments, like organisations, have a completely rational top priority, which is to survive. At both levels, the instigation and management of change are fundamental to that survival. To introduce change can be painful for both recipients and innovators. For this reason, the threat of conflict, as Handy (1985) has persuasively argued, has to be foreseen and avoided. In the health service, managers, par excellence, have to be diplomats. The advice that they have to give both to practitioners and to lay members of boards will show an awareness of the political demands on the organisation without appearing to support or to take issue with those demands. The political pragmatism of governments needs to be translated into organisational pragmatism by turning technically desirable options into politically feasible solutions.

Commissioning evaluation research

In order to assist the decision making process, health care service organisations commission external research bodies to carry out a formal evaluation of aspects of services and service provision. For example, one of the authors has been part of a team commissioned by a health care trust to assess the adequacy, take-up and quality of mental health services following the closure of a specialist hospital. All three authors have also carried out a three-year project evaluating the cost-effectiveness of multi-professional community based services designed to maintain vulnerable elderly people in their own homes rather than entering hospital or residential accommodation.

This formal evaluation adds to the repertoire of methods that can be applied in order to assess different aspects of organisational and staff performance, a topic dealt with in Chapter 4. Formal evaluation is a particular kind of social science research and, therefore, employs research designs, data collection methods and analytical criteria appropriate to the particular nature of the evaluation. Reference has already been made in Chapter 2 to key approaches to and models of evaluation. In this chapter we choose to concentrate on two particular aspects of formal evaluation: political and ethical matters. This is because the political and ethical contexts in which management decisions are located provide both limiting and helpful parameters for decision making. A second reason for pursuing this twofold perspective is that external evaluators themselves are not devoid of either political or ethical commitments and are likely to reflect this in their methodology and in their findings.

The politics of evaluation in the health care system

Essentially the study of politics is the study of power and how it is acquired and used. It is important in relation to evaluation in health care systems because those who control evaluation processes are likely to have a good deal of influence on the formulation of health policies. This is indicated in the model set out in Chapter 1 on page 4, by the arrow which goes from the 'evaluate' box to the 'input' box, a link that some refer to as the 'policy cycle' (Rist, 1995). In the 'evaluate' box itself there will be considerable impact from the model's central box (incrementalism, including Lindblom's (1959) 'partisan mutual adjustments') for, as Palumbo (1987) has argued, evaluations 'are inherently and unavoidably political' (p. 12). This is partly because there is no sustainable reason why evaluators should take the goals or objective of a policy or service as 'given' or 'good'. Objectives might be appropriate or inappropriate: for example, we would class Harold Shipman's objectives (see Chapter 5) as inappropriate and morally repugnant. We believe that it is a legitimate – indeed an important part of an evaluator's task to question the appropriateness of a service's objectives. It is therefore difficult, and often unwise, for evaluators to seek to be 'neutral'.

Power may be conceptualised in various ways (see, for example, Lukes, 1974; Hill, 1997). It may be seen as the ability:

- to get others to do what one wants them to do
- to do what one wants to do despite resistance from others
- to get people to want what one wants them to want
- to ensure that one's interests are served by a system or organisation

One of the difficulties faced by political scientists is how to find out who has most of the power in any system, be it an organisation, a city or a nation state. It might be that not only do we not know definitely who has the power but it is possible that we do not even know how to find out.

An early contribution to finding out 'who has power?' was the work of Hunter (1953) whose research method was based on asking people who they *thought* had most of the power. However, this study was criticised by Dahl (1957, 1961) who argued that it indicated who had a 'reputation' for having power which was not the same as actually having power itself. Dahl's 'decision making' approach involved studies of 'important' issues where there were disagreements (conflict) between people about what should be done. Actors whose preferences prevailed in such conflicting situations could, argued Dahl, be regarded as having decisive power. According to this view one thus 'needs to analyse concrete decisions involving actors pursuing different preferences. Careful study of these decisions is required before the distribution of power can be described adequately' (Hill, 1997, p. 38).

Bachrach & Baratz (1962) were unconvinced by Dahl's approach. They argued that studies of power should not be limited to actual behaviour and decision making as this would confine one's attention to issues that were clearly on the political agenda. It is possible that some people have the power to limit the scope of the political process to 'safe' issues (that is, issues that are innocuous to those with most of the power). This 'mobilisation of bias' (Schattschneider, 1960, p. 71) could help those with power to retain and use power by a process of 'non decision making'. Conflict is seen as less overt in the Bachrach and Baratz model than in the Dahl model in which it is clearly observable. In studying power, it is therefore important to study what does *not* happen as well as what *does* happen. Co-opting groups into the political arena might be one way in which 'non decision making' is exercised (Hill, 1997, p. 39).

The idea of the 'third dimension' of power was developed by Lukes (1974) in recognition of the fact that conflict is not necessarily a precondition of the exercise of power (as had been suggested by Dahl and by Bachrach & Baratz). Lukes argued that power could be used as a means of conflict avoidance by shaping people's preferences and perceptions. People's interests can thus be served or denied by the 'deep structure' of assumptions and embedded 'values' (see the central box in the model in Chapter 1) which influence policy processes in relatively subtle ways.

There are a number of models which seek to explain the distribution of power within the state. The principal models may be summarised as follows: pluralism; elite theory; ruling class theory; public choice theory; the 'third way', a representative and responsible government; party government; 'bureaucratic power' government; the technocratic view; and the administrative dispersion and diffusion view (Burch & Wood, 1983; Rhodes & Dunleavy, 1995; Hill, 1997; Budge *et al.*, 1998). We will discuss these below.

Pluralism

This model of largely decentralised or diffused power has been summarised by (Palfrey *et al.*, 1992, p. 37):

> Pluralists regard the State as a liberal representative democracy within which the competition for votes forces representatives to respond to the electorate's wishes. State bureaucracies which implement policies are seen as being responsive both to their political 'leaders' and to the public at large, especially when the electorate operate within interest groups which are depicted as the crucial components of political reality. Individuals express their preferences which are assumed to equate with their own best interests. Viewed from a pluralist perspective, political power is decentralised. . . . Consequently, no prevailing interest dominates the policy making process and competing interest

groups serve to maintain social equilibrium through a counterbalance of power.

A particularly useful contribution to pluralist theory, and especially the role of pressure groups, is the work of Richardson & Jordan (1979). In the context of the health care system the work of pressure groups may be seen in relation both to 'producer groups', such as the British Medical Association (BMA), Eckstein (1960), and the Royal College of Nursing (RCN); and to 'consumer groups', such as patient forums or MIND, the campaign group for the mentally ill.

Generally speaking, producer groups tend to have more influence in the political system than consumer groups do. In the case of the BMA, for example, an almost symbiotic relationships exists between that group and the Department of Health (Ham, 1992). Consumer groups, on the other hand, tend 'to have somewhat less influence, partly because their cooperation is usually not as significant for policy makers' (Ham, 1992, p. 114). Furthermore, consumer groups tend to have far fewer sanctions than do producer groups who can, for example, threaten to withdraw their cooperation and thus increase their influence.

Elite theory

This model has been summarised as follows (Palfrey *et al.*, 1992, p. 38):

> Here power is not decentralised as the pluralists claim, but is concentrated in the hands of an elite minority, e.g. individuals who move in each other's circles, including the senior Civil Service, Government, family connections, the professions, company directorships, public schools and Oxbridge. Elite theorists suggest there is little or no competition to constrain the power of the elite, and that most people (the non-elite) are acquiescent and unorganised. There is a consistent bias in the policy process of state bureaucracies in favour of elite groups, and much power is concentrated in bureaucracies which are largely under the control of the elite groups. . . . There are many

interests (often 'concealed' because of the way in which the policy process operates), which are unrepresented, or under-represented, in the political system; e.g. the unemployed, the chronically sick and handicapped, and the elderly.

Several studies into power in the NHS have concluded that the elite model provides the most useful explanation of how power operates within the health care system. For example, it has been suggested (Haywood & Alaszewski, 1980; Ham, 1981; Harrison *et al.*, 1990) that the medical profession has retained decisive control over the allocation of resources by the maintenance of an ideological framework within which other employees work; this is achieved by the retention of a high degree of clinical autonomy and a continued emphasis on a medical model of health, that is a model which is individualistic and disease based, as opposed to a more collective approach which seeks to prevent the causes of ill health – poor diet, cigarette smoking, lack of exercise, environmental pollution, workplace conditions, unemployment, poverty and poor housing.

The ruling class theory (or Marxist theory)

This model has been summarised as follows (Palfrey *et al.*, 1992, pp. 38–9):

> Capitalist societies . . . are those which are divided into two economic classes based on the ownership and control of the means of production (wealth) – the bourgeoisie (the ruling class) and the proletariat. According to a Marxist interpretation, 'class conflict' is inevitable and as a result of policy processes, benefits consistently go to the ruling class whose interests are served by the state; e.g. the state ensures the maintenance/survival of the economic system in the following ways:
>
> - *government economic policy*: e.g. subsidies to industry
> - *reproduction of the labour force*: e.g. the 'welfare state' provides a healthy, trained, housed, docile labour force

- *ideology*: an ideological supremacy is sustained by way of the education system, the mass media and the family
- *repression*: the state has a monopoly of 'legitimate' violence (the police and the military)
- *the legal system*: e.g. property rights are guaranteed otherwise capitalists would not invest
- *the monetary system*: the means of exchange and orderly international trade
- *foreign policy*: e.g. diplomatic relations with the Arab oil-producing countries during the early 1970s

The state will not necessarily always favour the ruling class: e.g. in order to maintain the legitimacy of the system, it may be necessary to allow some gains to the proletariat (e.g. the welfare state). By 'buying off' social unrest, the state can thus demonstrate that it operates in everyone's interests – a pretence of neutrality.

Marxist theory has been used by several analysts to explain the way that capitalism influences health and health care in certain ways (for example, Navarro, 1978 and Doyal & Pennell, 1979). It can be argued that health problems are created by the way in which the capitalist system works, for example: by the way in which industry is organised (creating pollution, health and safety problems and the creation of stress by machine paced work); by the products of industry (unhealthy foods, cigarettes and alcohol) and by the creation of ill health through poverty/economic inequalities. The argument can be extended to the way in which health problems are 'solved', for example: the emphasis on getting people back to work ('cure' services given more resources than 'care' services); the 'individualising' of health problems (the medical model as opposed to more collective health promotion policies) and the creation of profits for pharmaceutical firms, manufacturers of medical equipment and building contractors.

The conclusion reached by some 'ruling class' theorists is that the health care system, therefore, mainly serves the interests of industry and the capitalists who own most of it. However, it could be argued that the problems highlighted are not those of capitalism per se, but of industrialisation.

Public choice theory and the 'new right'

Public choice theory rejects the above models and stresses the importance of individual choice (an economics model of the utility-maximising individual, i.e. individuals maximise satisfaction to themselves). The emphasis is on a neo-liberal view which is hostile to the welfare state as institutions which impose an unsustainable burden on the state. Processes and structures (e.g. planning and large bureaucratic organisations), essential to a welfare state, are criticised as being a threat to liberty and freedom.

Central to public choice theory are the notions:

(1)   that the state should have only a limited role
(2)   that individuals know better than the state bureaucracies what is good for them
(3)   that the private provision of services, including health and social care, is nearly always better than provision of services by the state. This is so because of the following inter-linked arguments.

Many of those who support this view claim that some groups (e.g. the trade unions) have been too powerful, and that the whole political system can sometimes be out of control in that there can be an 'overload' of demands on Government because of public expectations, increasing bureaucracy and the increased activities of pressure groups. The approach of public choice theorists to health care is likely to be to leave to individuals the responsibility to make provision for their own needs (for example, by way of private provision or insurance).

Those who support a right wing approach to managing health care systems are likely to favour approaches which make full use of competitive forces as a way of increasing the efficiency of the system. This was the case when the Thatcher Government introduced its internal market reforms (DHSS, 1989) based on the work of Enthoven (1985).

The 'third way'

This has been associated with Tony Blair's 'New Labour'. The view seeks to find what some people see as a 'middle way' between traditional views of left wing politics (with its emphasis on planning, public service and altruism) and right wing politics (with its neo-liberal emphasis on markets and freedom for individuals to pursue self interests). Those who support the 'third way' are often advocates of appropriate balances between seemingly contradictory principles, for example, the need for *national* standards and priorities (such as the guidance from the National Institute for Clinical Excellence and the development of national service frameworks) and the need for responsiveness to *locally* defined needs and priorities, as when primary care trusts are expected to assess local health care needs and plan local services to meet those needs. Other 'compromises' would include the adoption of appropriate doses of rational planning together with market-tested efficiencies.

A representative and responsible government (the Westminster model)

In this model the distinction between policy and administration (the execution of policy decisions) is very clear. Politicians are assumed to make policy, and administrators (Civil Servants, health care managers, local government officials etc.) are expected to implement it. The model emphasises:

(1) elections and electoral systems
(2) the Cabinet (drawn mainly from elected members of the House of Commons)
(3) parliament (and local authorities in the case of local government) controlling the 'executive'
(4) the Crown

This model is deceptive. It is the view that is held by many politicians and by large parts of the general public. Yet questions can be raised about its validity in practice. For example, to what extent does the legislature (Parliament) actually control the executive (the Government) in practice? Where a party has a large majority in the House of Commons – as the Labour Party enjoyed in the years following its substantial general election victory in 1997 – it will often find it can carry through its will in promoting new policies and laws with little effective opposition. The debate about the introduction of 'foundation hospitals' in England in 2003 may be seen as a recent example of what Hailsham termed an 'elective dictatorship' (Hailsham, 1976).

Party government

This is similar to the above view but in this case the key institutions are the political parties rather than elected assemblies.

> It is political parties that mediate the public's opinion, which they can fuse into broad policy proposals; it is the political parties that control the operations of the assembly. Parties thus predominate in the formulation of policy, and control the policy process.
>
> (Burch & Wood, 1983, p. 33)

The role of parties and their commitments was exemplified by the introduction of compulsory competitive tendering (CCT) for 'hotel services' – such as cleaning, laundry and catering – in hospitals, a policy which was introduced in the 1980s by the Conservative party and strongly opposed by the Labour party and most of the trade union movement.

'Bureaucratic power' government

This view focuses on government machinery (e.g. ministries and local government departments) rather than assemblies and parties. In this model it is the paid officials (civil servants, local government officers, etc.) or bureaucrats who have the power, not the politicians. This model was nicely illustrated in the BBC TV series 'Yes Minister' in which the often hapless minister would usually be out-manoeuvred by his manipulative and urbane permanent secretary.

As Ham (1992, p. 107) has pointed out, civil servants have considerably more influence over policy processes than suggested in many textbook accounts. Politicians can, and sometimes do, get their way, as was the case when Richard Crossman at the DHSS succeeded in establishing the Hospital Advisory Service in 1969. On many issues, however, they often have more difficulty and 'have to bargain, cajole and compromise before they get their way' (Ham, 1992, p. 107).

A number of misgivings have been expressed (as in the BBC TV Panorama programme broadcast on 29 June 2003) about the relationship between targets, especially those relating to patients' waiting times and health care professionals' opinions on clinical priorities. For example, it is suggested that high priority patients (from a clinical need perspective) can sometimes be put 'on hold' in order to avoid additional patients having to wait longer than the time allowed by a threshold waiting target. Health care managers often see themselves as being under intense pressure to achieve these bureaucratically imposed targets in order to achieve a high 'star' rating for their hospital trust. This point is further discussed later in the chapter.

The technocratic view

Here the emphasis is on professionals or technical experts (e.g. economists, scientists) who, it is argued, are the best people to make key decisions because of the technical issues involved. The tradition in the UK, however, is to have such specialists 'on tap' rather than 'on top' It is usually career civil servants with a generalist education who are 'on top' of the official side of Government departments. Nevertheless the role of technical experts clearly becomes more important when the Government needs professional advice from medical officers and consultants when responding to health crises such as BSE, food poisoning events and the SARS (severe acute respiratory syndrome) scare in 2003.

The administrative dispersion and diffusion view

The view here is that many problems are now so complex that no one institution can realistically hope to deal with them effectively. The emphasis is therefore on recognising fragmentation and on inter-organisational collaboration, partnership and networking. This is an issue which we examined in Chapter 2 in relation to problems requiring inter-organisational collaboration in relation to health care.

The above models are not mutually exclusive (the boundaries between some of them are very blurred) but the models differ in the emphasis they give to the various institutions of the state. There is no 'correct' model or version of reality. As Allison (1971) demonstrated, various models are alternative ways of seeing realities from different viewpoints for what one sees depends on where one stands and on which viewing instrument one uses. Models are more or less useful in terms of the ways they can help to explain what is going on, how and why.

Structural interests

An analysis which is based on an elite model is the idea of structural interests developed by Alford (1975). Structural interests are different from 'interest groups' in that structural interests either do not need to organise themselves (because current arrangements already benefit them) or they find great difficulty in effectively organising themselves into influential interest groups, as in the case of the most poorly resourced groups. Alford offers a threefold classification of structural interests:

- *dominant structural interests*: for example, the 'professional monopolisers' like medical practitioners
- *challenging structural interests*: for example, corporate rationalisers such as planners, managers, administrators and researchers who are 'challenging the fundamental interests of professional monopolisers and exerting increasing influence over the production and distribution of health care' (Palfrey, 2000, p. 23)
- *repressed structural interests*: for example, the community population which finds that it is unable to have any real influence

As Ham points out: 'dominant interests are served by existing social, economic and political institutions and therefore only need to be active when their interests are challenged' (1992, p. 223). In Chapter 2 we referred to the way in which health care managers have, to some extent, challenged the professional autonomy and power of medical practitioners. Nevertheless, despite increasing challenges by corporate rationalisers, the medical profession still retains decisive influence over the allocation of resources within the NHS.

People's views about which is the most useful political model for analysing power and politics in the NHS will vary, but whatever shape power relationships take they feed into the modified systems model which was set out in Chapter 1 on page 4, as a set of 'inputs'. For example, a new Government policy on evaluating hospitals such as the star rating system, or the creation of new institutions, such as the Audit Commission in 1983 or the Commission for Health Care Audit and Inspection in 2004, will shape the way in which managers and professionals undertake their work within the health care system. Knowledge of the political influences is therefore helpful in understanding why and how the system and its sub-systems perform as they do.

At the organisational level, health care managers commonly rely on their 'position power' (French & Raven, 1968). This is the power that managers have over others because of the position they occupy in the hierarchical structure of the trust or other health care agency. For most people, if the manager asks for something to be done, and they think it is a reasonable instruction (for example, it is legal and ethical) then they will usually comply even if they disagree with the decision. They might query it but often people think 'I think the managers are wrong here, but they have to carry the can so we'll go along with it'. This is commonly underpinned by 'resource power' (French & Raven, 1968) which is the power exerted by someone who has control over resources which are highly valued by the people they are trying to influence. There have to be three elements present for this to work:

- the person has to have actual control over the resource in question (merely to *claim* the control is not enough)
- the resource must be highly valued by the target persons
- the target persons must have no other source of the resource in question (i.e. the target needs to be highly dependent on the person trying to exercise influence)

Within health care organisations these two forms of power, based on position and resource dependency, are commonly held together in relation to a particular relationship because managers usually have more control over scarce resources (including the budget, office space and the operation of staff appraisal systems) than do staff who are accountable to them. However, there is a form of organisational power which is more problematic for many managers within health care systems. This is the power that health care professionals, such as medical practitioners, nurses and professionals allied to medicine (PAMs), often have in clinical situations. It is the power they have because 'outsiders' (such as managers, patients and patients' families) often defer to the opinions of professionals who are perceived as having highly valued clinical expertise. Outsiders often defer to professionals because they fear the consequences of not doing so.

One of the interesting aspects of this kind of 'expert power' (French & Raven, 1968) is that, unlike position power, it can operate in various directions in the hierarchical structure of health care agencies: downwards, upwards, sideways or diagonally. It is not reliant on the 'power holder' being near the top of the official hierarchy. The position may be further complicated by the presence of what French & Raven (1968) call 'referent power', that is the power exercised by the personal magnetism or charisma of particular individuals.

Yukl (1998) has built on French & Raven's classification in a very explicit way and has offered ideas about how one can increase, maintain and use the different forms of power within organisations. In this way managers and professionals may extend their influence over, for example, how a particular policy or service should be evaluated in relation to the criteria to be used and how they should be weighted. This can influence the results of an evaluation and therefore the ways in which the policy or service may be developed in the future.

Accountability and control

An important process by which power may be exercised is that of accountability, which concerns the ways in which managers and professionals can be called to account for what they have done, how and why. In any hierarchical structure authority goes 'downwards' and accountability (or responsibility) goes 'upwards'. Accountability is a particularly important issue in public sector management for, as Hudson points out (in Hill, 1997, p. 398), 'accountability is the link between bureaucracy and democracy'. There are four important dimensions of accountability (Elcock & Haywood, 1980) which help to map out the political influences, including control, within and between organisations, as follows.

Location of accountability

Traditionally ministers were held accountable for everything done by their departments. If necessary the minister was expected to resign. But in recent years this expectation has been modified because it is thought unreasonable to expect ministers to be responsible for *all* errors made by civil servants. However:

> the problems caused by the increase in the size of departments were highlighted by the enquiry into the failure of the DTI to avert the collapse of the Vehicle and General Insurance Company in 1971. In its evidence, the Department stated that well under 1% of its business was referred to Ministers. Largely for this reason, the tribunal exonerated all the Ministers and laid the blame on . . . a named civil servant'.
>
> (Brown & Steel, 1979, pp. 130–31)

Furthermore, select committees have established the right to cross examine civil servants as well as ministers. Accountability has thus become more 'shared'. Nevertheless an essential element of evaluation, performance management and clinical governance is to be able to identify who is going to be held accountable for processes (means) and performance (ends). The public generally, and specific clients of health services, understandably wish to know who they can hold accountable for what is done and what is achieved and what is not achieved.

Direction of accountability

Normally managers are accountable to their 'line manager'. But issues which can confuse the direction of accountability include professional status, trade unionism, consumerism, and organisation structures; for example, to whom is a Government accountable – the House of Commons, taxpayers, the electorate, the community at large, the courts, the users of services, the mass media. Sometimes staff believe that they have a wider responsibility than to their direct 'managers', e.g. do civil servants have a wider responsibility to Parliament and the public if they think that a minister is misleading Parliament? In a complex system like the NHS, managers and professionals commonly find themselves facing in several directions. They may be accountable to a range of people and agencies. Life in a modern health care system is rarely a comfortable one.

Content of accountability

The creation of the Audit Commission in the early 1980s increased the range of matters for which managers and professionals in the public sector would be held accountable. Before that time managers were accountable for acting with probity, for example to ensure that money was spent honestly for its intended purpose. Notions of 'value for money' mean that managers are now also accountable for efficient and effective performance. In recent years this has meant that managers and professionals in the NHS are expected to achieve a range of targets, many of which relate in various ways to waiting times, which are not always wholeheartedly welcomed by those within the system.

The increase in 'target culture', which can sometimes focus unduly on those things which are relatively easy to quantify, is thought by some to divert resources away from more important long-term service developments. In a letter published in the *Guardian* on 10 June 2003, James Strachan (the chairman of the Audit Commission) raised three important questions about NHS targets:

- do they focus properly on outcomes for service users or just on processes?

- are there too many to be effective?
- have people wrongly started to treat them as ends in themselves and not what they really are: tools for improvement?

We believe that Governments need to address these questions carefully when deciding how to take forward their future policies on the imposition of goals, objectives and targets. Accountability and 'chains of command' are important, but so is an appropriate degree of autonomy for managers and health care professionals.

Mechanisms of control

Control is achieved by the ability to hold people accountable. Control may be exercised by the control of scarce resources or by the law. The law also has an important part to play in various ways; for example, professional staff are accountable to the public, to the law, to their clients (the possibility of being sued in civil law), to their employers (by way of their contract of employment) and their profession (through professional conduct committees).

The four dimensions of accountability can be summarised thus: *who* is accountable *to whom*, for *what* and *how*? In any public sector organisation such as the NHS, managers and professionals need to have clear answers to this four dimensional question.

In Chapter 2 we discussed some aspects of the changing power relationships between medical practitioners and managers within health care settings. What our discussion of power and accountability suggests is that the various stakeholders in health care settings (and in health care evaluations in particular) have different degrees of different forms of power and are enmeshed in various structures of accountability. They will have different priorities, and their ability to influence health policy processes will be contingent on both visible and less obvious forces within the health care system.

Medical practitioners, for example, have traditionally had most of the power in the health care system (Harrison *et al.*, 1990), though Ong *et al.* (1997) have offered an alternative insight into the 'doctors versus managers' tension. They point out that the debate commonly centres on whether it is the managers who are gaining ground or whether it is doctors. These two models now need to give way to a third model which 'allows for a more dynamic understanding of the role of hospital doctors' (Ong *et al.*, 1997, p. 91).

The concerns that consultants have in relation to resources, quality of care, clinical judgement and in relation to managerial perspectives on cost cutting and maximising income mean that the thinking of consultants and managers tend to converge. Doctors, therefore, are increasingly working with managers or are becoming managers, albeit in a part-time or transient capacity in many cases. The need to appear 'attractive' (in terms of cost and quality of services) to those who commission services (for example, primary care trusts) tends to encourage cooperation between doctors and managers in a shared need to gain support from commissioners. 'Doctors will, therefore, engage in short or medium-term alliances with managers in order to safeguard their [position]' (Ong *et al.*, 1997, p. 92).

One of the key political issues that emerges in the context of evaluation in the NHS is whether evaluators should adopt an openly ideological mission to alter the imbalance of power between decision makers and largely repressed social groups. On the one hand one could argue (see, for example, Palfrey & Thomas, 1999, p. 59) that agencies, such as Government departments, that commission evaluations should be urged by evaluators to recognise the legitimate interests of all stakeholders in contributing to the evaluation process. On the other hand, one could go further (as we prefer) and accept that a comprehensive range of multiple stakeholder criteria is essential for assessing the value of particular programmes, because the logic of evaluation demands a pluralistic approach (Smith & Cantley, 1985). Whether evaluators ought to go as far as acting as assertive advocates of social justice is a moot point. At the very least we would argue that there is a need for evaluators to understand the political system in which each evaluation is undertaken.

Evaluators, be they managers or health care professionals, thus need to address questions such as:

- in whose interests is this particular programme supposed to work?
- who decided on the goals of the programme (goal based evaluation tends to be politically biased towards those goals favoured by dominant groups)?
- who will select the evaluative criteria to be used in the evaluation?
- who will decide on how the criteria will be weighted?
- who will control the data collection process?
- what kind of approach will be used for the collection and analysis of data?
- who are the key stakeholders in relation to the programme in question?
- who will control the final report and the extent to which its recommendations are acted upon?

There are those who argue that the role of evaluators should be politically neutral. We believe that this position is untenable for any one decision (for example, in relation to what data are to be collected or what criteria are to be used in undertaking an evaluation) will tend to favour, wittingly or unwittingly, one group more than another. As Guba & Lincoln (1989) and others have argued, we cannot safely assume that evaluators can be and should be politically neutral. Evaluations are inherently and inevitably political. The important thing is for evaluators to be aware of the political context of any evaluation and to perform their work ethically and with transparent values. It is the politically significant issue of values that is emphasised in the central box in the model which we outlined in Chapter 1 on page 4, and to which we now turn.

Ethical perspectives on health care management

An evaluative approach to health care management admits the likelihood that there is room for improvement in various aspects of the organisation's functioning: in its structure, its strategy, its financial risk management, its systems of clinical governance and in its overall corporate governance. As we have discussed in Chapter 4, there is a range of devices for monitoring and reviewing performance which are integral to the management process. Formal evaluation, however, involves a longer-term and frequently more detailed assessment of the organisation's performance in specific areas of operation.

Writing in 1980 Sieber commented that 'there is virtually no literature on the ethics of program evaluation' (Sieber, 1980, p. 52). In the succeeding years, in the UK and the USA, this particular deficiency has remained, with one or two exceptions (Bulmer, 1982; Punch, 1986; Chambers *et al.*, 1992; Cheetham *et al.*, 1992). In evaluation research, in which judgements are often made about the effectiveness and cost effectiveness of certain policy interventions, a clear exposition of the value-stances of key participants should be essential since opinions about what constitutes 'success' are likely to be rooted in ideological as well as pragmatic interests (Palfrey & Thomas, 1996).

One of the primary ethical considerations in evaluating organisational performance is the extent to which patients are invited to express their views on aspects of a service of which they have had some experience. Any research which seeks to involve patients will have to go before the relevant ethics committee for approval. This process emphasises the need to conduct research in a manner that does not put patients at risk, will not breach codes of confidentiality and which treats them with respect. In this regard, the ethics of evaluation are entirely compatible with codes of ethics for managers and for all professional staff working in the health service.

However, there could be a different emphasis between external evaluators and health care managers in the role of patients in the evaluation. Patient satisfaction surveys remain the staple method for seeking the opinions of patients and ex-patients on a hospital's 'performance'. Yet their construction is often the work of persons other than patients themselves. Our examination of many patient satisfaction questionnaires, for example, reveals a mix of poorly constructed questions, an excessive number of items and little opportunity to attach ratings or scores to various aspects of the patient's experience. In short, they can be accused of adopting, in both research and ideological terms, an unethical inclination towards professional/managerial bias.

There is not only a compelling logic to engage patients or former patients in the construction of patient satisfaction questionnaires, but an ethical dimension, because to exclude patients from this particular evaluation enterprise is to announce implicitly that managers and professionals are quite happy to colonise patients' areas of expertise but that the converse would not be acceptable.

Gillon (1994) listed a number of ethical factors that were relevant to the practice of medicine. They are: honesty, equity, impartiality, respect and a high level of competence. Confidentiality could, of course, be added to the list. We shall comment on each of these attributes with regard to their applicability to health care management.

Honesty

- Agencies that commission evaluation studies – health authorities, health care trusts, primary care groups/local health boards should be explicit about their willingness and capacity to implement changes if the results of the evaluation indicate that such changes are desirable.
- Commissioning agencies should be specific at the outset regarding the feasibility of change within earmarked or designated budgets.
- Commissioning agencies should enable external evaluators to decide on the most appropriate research designs and data collection methods in order to produce valid data. There should also be open debate about the criteria to be used in evaluating a particular programme or service activity.

Equity

- This ethical principle involves the concepts of impartiality and natural justice: that people with similar needs ought to be treated in a similar way.

- In the context of service evaluation, this principle in action would require the evaluator to include the views of all principal stakeholders and interest groups.
- Not only will the evaluation include all stakeholders and interest groups, but their contributions to the evaluation will be considered to be of potentially equal validity and relevance.

Impartiality

- In a sense, this ethical principle is a means towards achieving equity. An impartial evaluator will treat each contributing perspective with equal respect. There will be no predisposition to value the opinions or assessments of any particular contributor more highly than any other.
- Although the evaluator can never be a completely neutral observer and interpreter, there has to be an attempt to keep an open mind about the evidence to be gathered and about its meaning. There should be no attempt to prove a prior hypothesis or ideological commitment; only to sift as comprehensive a set of data as possible and draw logical inferences.
- An awareness of what might be anticipated as comfortable or acceptable conclusions as far as management is concerned should not compromise the integrity of the research findings.

Respect

- This aspect relates to questions of equity. Even though (ex-)patients, for example, might have little or no knowledge of or insights into the priorities attached by physicians, politicians or managers to health service provision, they have a distinctive expertise in what it is like to be a patient.
- Respect for people means that statements about the importance of involving 'the public' in judgements about the quality of health services are more than political rhetoric. The policy of patient and public participation is

embedded in the organisation's mechanisms for seeking and acting upon 'external' critiques.

- Respect also implies mutuality rather than necessarily consensus: an agreed tolerance of differing views.

Adherence to high levels of competence

Physicians, as managers, work within an ethical frame of reference. Florence Nightingale's reputed statement that the primary aim of nursing was 'to do the sick no harm' exemplifies the moral imperative of *non-maleficence*. Its associated, more positive aspiration is *beneficence* – the use of resources and knowledge in order to provide maximum possible benefit to patients. The Hippocratic oath binds members of the medical profession to adhere to a strict code of conduct which places the interest of the patient at the heart of medical practice. The lengthy period of education which precedes qualification as a medical practitioner and the control over entry to and dismissal from the medical register by professional medical associations testifies to a concern with maintaining high standards of competence. Departure from such standards, through negligence or wilful deviation from the principles of the Hippocratic oath, constitutes a serious breach of ethics.

But while medical practitioners are dedicated to the observance of confidentiality on an individual patient level, when they assume the role of manager in various health care contexts, the need to display a commitment to openness is paramount. Health care managers are expected to work to high levels of competence within a clear ethical framework. The Nolan Committee report (1995) laid down seven principles of public life that apply to all staff and non-executive board members within the NHS and other public bodies, such as local authorities. They are:

- *selflessness*: decisions are to be taken solely in terms of the public interest and not in order to gain a financial or other material benefit for oneself, family or friends
- *integrity*: there must be no financial or other obligation to outside individuals or organisations that might influence members or staff in the performance of their official duties

- *objectivity*: in carrying out public business, including making appointments to posts, awarding contracts or recommending individuals for rewards or benefits, choices should be made on merit
- *accountability*: decision makers are accountable to the public and must submit themselves to whatever scrutiny is appropriate to their office
- *openness*: decisions made and actions taken must be as open as possible with information restricted only when the wider public interest demands it
- *honesty*: there is a duty to declare any private interests relating to one's public duties and to take steps to resolve any conflicts arising in a way that protects the public interest
- *leadership*: these principles should be promoted and supported by leadership and examples

Summarising the above seven principles is the notion of *probity*. An extremely important aspect of this overriding principle is the efficient and effective stewardship of public funds. Financial management demands a combination of high ethical and professional standards towards the implementation of an effective risk management policy.

Potential for conflict

The seven guiding principles expressed by the Nolan Committee for ensuring ethical conduct within public services are hardly contestable. Yet adherence to all of them does not preclude the possibility of tension and even conflict between stakeholders in evaluating and planning resources. Health economists, for example, have argued the case for the 'collective ethic' to be placed above the 'individual ethic' in the context of decisions relating to where finite resources should be allocated (Maynard, 1991). This exposition of neo-utilitarianism depends for its validity on an increasing body of knowledge about the health impact and costs of certain treatments for particular health conditions – the evidence-based approach discussed in Chapters 3 and 5.

The greatest good of the greatest number is an ethically attractive health care objective; one that emphasises the strong moral imperative to use resources where they will produce maximum benefit. In a television documentary screened at a time when the UK Government was about to implement a purchaser-provider split of functions within the NHS, the reference point was the Oregon system of deciding which health care services the state was prepared to subsidise. This radical attempt to involve the public in devising a list of treatments and conditions that would or would not be supported by public funds remains a virtually unique example of explicit rationing and prioritising of resources. This approach has not been replicated in any other state in the USA but remains popular with the Oregon people. A recent attempt, for example, by a political faction to expand the system to one approaching a quasi-NHS system failed to gain enough support to change the status quo (Oregon website, 2003).

The success of the Oregon system is that it has managed to combine improved access to services for poorer people previously excluded from certain subsidised treatments while reducing demand for certain services, many of which were previously subsidised. The public, by being involved in decisions about which conditions should be included on the list, have made a collective ethical and financial judgement. The decision about who is allowed or denied access to public health care services rests on a fundamental value judgement about the nature of health itself. If, as many influential clinicians in Oregon argued, health is regarded as a commodity in the same sense as a car or washing machine, then it follows that the corresponding health care system will not be founded on the principle of equity. Nevertheless, in the context of the USA, Oregon has probably gone as far as it is possible to go along the road to an alternative to an almost exclusively insurance-based funding of health care services.

While many economists and health care managers in the UK are likely to find the collective ethic a more persuasive economic doctrine than currently prevails, the tension between the collective and the individual as the focus of resource allocation decisions can be experienced in the day to day practice of clinician-managers. For example, one paediatrician in the documentary referred to above, explained that given the choice between carrying out expensive procedures for keeping alive very underweight babies and spending money on educating mothers-to-be about ways to prevent or reduce the possibility of giving birth to low-weight babies, he would spend the money on the preventive care. Yet, in his words, 'it would take forcible restraint' to prevent him providing the best possible care to whichever baby was set before him. In the context of the collective and individual ethics debate, to explain to a parent that their child will have to die for the public good may be both ethically sound and morally repugnant.

The definition of ethics offered by Parker (1988) as 'using the tools of reason to generate rules which should guide our judgement in particular and general circumstances' appears to ignore the possibility that different rules dictated by different rational stances might operate in a clash between the particular and the general. Green (2001) argues that managers lack guidelines on how to incorporate an understanding of ethics into their decision making processes but her discussion is limited to the issue of suicide and references to the key ethical tenets propounded by a selective number of famous philosophers. Whether it is necessary for health care managers to know that Kant's categorical imperative was that we treat people as ends in themselves and not as means to an end or that Aristotle believed that each citizen had a duty to honour obligations to the community, is dubious.

The philosopher Alasdair Macintyre has pointed out that questions of ends are questions of values 'and on values reason is silent' (Macintyre, 1985, p. 26). Bureaucratic rationality is the rationality, he contends, of matching means to ends economically and efficiently. He further argues that 'conflict between rival values cannot be rationally settled' (p. 26). One must simply choose between parties, classes, causes, ideals. Macintyre's view of managers is that they treat ends as given and as outside their scope. In their role as manager, they are unable to engage in moral debate. Their task is to restrict themselves to the realms in which rational agreement is possible – that is, from their point of view, to the realms of fact, of means and of measurable effectiveness.

Effectiveness as an ethical concept

Macintyre (1985) asserts that we are not accustomed to doubt the effectiveness of managers in achieving what they set out to achieve and we are equally unaccustomed to think of effectiveness as a distinctively *moral* concept, to be classed with such ideas as rights or utilities. Managers themselves, he continues, conceive of themselves as morally neutral characters whose skills enable them to devise the most efficient means of achieving whatever end is proposed. However, there remains the question of the nature of the ends themselves and the ways in which managers try to ensure that those ends are achieved. According to Macintyre, the notion and assumption of effectiveness are used to sustain and extend the authority and power of managers and this imputation of effectiveness derives from a misplaced belief in managers' 'expertise'.

In attempting to demolish the credibility of managers possessing specialised knowledge which enables them to exert considerable influence within bureaucratic organisations, Macintyre, in effect, is discounting any evidence base to justify managerial decisions. Managers' claims to expertise rests on the supposed 'existence of a domain of morally neutral fact' accessible to a manager and on the capacity to deduce from 'law-like generalisations' that 'if an event or state of affairs of a certain type were to occur . . . some other event or state of affairs of some specific kind would result' (p. 77). Both claims mirror those made by the natural sciences and it is not surprising, argues Macintyre, that the term 'management science' should have been coined.

Macintyre's analysis of the means by which managers have acquired power and authority follows closely the central thesis of Weber's discourse on the rise of bureaucracy (Weber, 1947). It is also redolent of the thinking of Foucault (1973) and of Illich (1976) in their exposition of the evolution of medical dominance in the arena of health and health care.

In the view of these writers, managers and doctors have skilfully woven about themselves an aura of specialist expertise and knowledge that equips them to attain positions of considerable dominance within large organisations such as the NHS. With the advent of managerialism during the reorganisation of the NHS in the 1980s, the traditional monopoly of clinicians to decide where resources should be spent and on whom was challenged. The rise of the manager within the NHS and the emergence of management consultancy as a growth industry in both the commercial and public sectors suggests that there is, indeed, a scientific basis to management activities and that, consequently, managers have a *right* to be heavily involved in strategic decision making.

In one sense, therefore, the relentless commitment in many countries to producing hard evidence for clinical decisions has been influenced by the recognition that clinical decisions relating to diagnosis and treatment are not necessarily scientific: that the clinical knowledge base is not all that the medical profession would have us believe and that in a health care system unable to cope with increasing demand, we can no longer afford to allocate scarce resources on decisions based on clinical 'expertise' alone. Interestingly, the explicit claims of 'management' to be a science and, by implication, that managers have, by dint of being managers, specialist skills has led to recent and current debate about the need for evidence-based management, as we have noted in Chapter 3.

Criteria for evaluating health care services take on an ethical dimension according to the predominant values of the particular stakeholder. Doctors regard efficacy as the ultimate objective in a hierarchy of three major principles: to comfort; to relieve; to cure. Health economists are likely to rank efficiency as a key moral principle because this links positive effects of clinical interventions with the costs of generating those effects and waste of public funds is ethically indefensible. Managers, on the other hand, will probably regard effectiveness – achieving stated ends – as the rational and moral justification of their role. Yet we return to the question of what constitutes 'effectiveness' and, in Chapter 3, we have argued that this term is now largely determined and defined by agencies of Government within the UK through national service frameworks, prioritised spending areas and a multiplicity of targets. In this respect, Macintyre's rather searing attribution of what he terms a 'moral fiction' to managers' deceptive behaviour, appears less persuasive in the current situation within the NHS. On the other hand, Easton's description of policy making as the 'allocation of values' (Easton, 1965) seems particularly applicable at a time when economy, efficiency and effectiveness (with equity sometimes added) have been stipulated as the political priorities for evaluating health services and when 'quality' as almost a moral slogan, can be defined as the synthesis of the first three 'E's.

Ethical issues in allocating resources

Perhaps the most defining aspect of the role of managers within the health service relates to the allocation of resources to different treatments, health conditions and individual patients. The rise of managerialism in the NHS was predicated on a belief by successive Conservative Governments in the 1980s and 1990s that managers would be more likely to reduce wastage and enhance efficiency than members of the medical profession acting as a corporate group of decision makers. This assumption arose out of a political commitment to the transfer of management modes of operating in the commercial business sector to the publicly funded, not-for-profit NHS. It was felt that a more dispassionate, hardnosed approach to prioritising would create a health service that placed resources where they would be most cost-effective. In essence, therefore, the *value base* on which management practice was founded was to confront that shared by medical practitioners.

Loughlin (1998) presents a rigorous critique of the managerial perspective, bolstered by the claims of health economists, that prioritising decisions can be justified on grounds of efficient deployment of limited resources. Loughlin finds the espousal of QALYs, as an appropriate and morally acceptable method for making judgements on who gets what, to be a spuriously quantitative rationale for denying care to people who could benefit from it. In order to make 'rational' decisions on complex matters of resource allocation, Loughlin asserts that health care managers often view themselves as 'guardians' of the public interest. In the face of scarcity, managers are charged to 'lead, develop, control and evaluate' the work of professional carers (Wall, 1989). This responsibility rests on definitions – or, at least, interpretations of 'need'. One view of 'need', attractive to those who hold to an economically pragmatic perspective, is 'the capacity to benefit' from a particular service (Coast *et al.*, 1996, p. 145). This can then be developed into an Oregon-type formula that uses QALYs to compare projected benefits (length of benefit/length of life plus quality of life) among contesting claimants for treatment.

Loughlin argues that the adoption of QALYs as a means of *measuring* health status and health gain is a specious device since there can be such divergent opinions about what constitutes 'quality of life'. The Oregon attempt to aggregate public opinion in order to produce a seeming consensus cannot be regarded as authentic. Furthermore, according to Wall (1989), 'choosing ways to spend [health] resources is not a rational process. It is largely influenced by assumptions and powerful groups, all as potent as they are non-rational', p. 101. Despite the involvement of the public in Oregon, we know that some of their rankings appeared rather eccentric to the medical practitioners on the State's Steering Group and were relocated as a result. (Coast *et al.*, 1996).

Wall (1994) has also rejected the idea that rationality has anything to do with management. If his contention holds true, is it meaningful to discuss evaluative approaches to management? Can there be a rational underpinning of resource allocation decisions? Loughlin (1998) refers to 'the brutality and injustice in any rationing procedure' and maintains that acknowledging the need to ration and prioritise resources presumes a social world that cannot be altered: that scarcity is inherent in the NHS and therefore inescapable.

The natural corollary of this line of reasoning is that in a truly equitable and 'moral' health care system, resources would be infinite or at least the capacity to shape demand in line with finite resources would be achievable. Neither position is tenable unless we are to adopt an even more ethically 'brutal' policy of 'equitable rationing' in its true sense and allocate a fixed amount of money per citizen, regardless of wealth, in order to gain access to health care on a kind of voucher system. This would not take into account different severity of need in terms of life-saving treatments, alleviation of chronic symptoms, rehabilitative and palliative care services. There is surely a moral position between the greatest good of the greatest number and the ethics of treating patients whatever the short or long-term benefits are likely to be.

It is easy to attempt to demolish the credibility of QALYs as a tool for measuring potential health benefits as a result of medical interventions. Of course 'quality of life' is an elusive concept, subjective at best, meaningless at worst. However, there is undeniably a need to manage human and financial resources having regard to the demands and perspectives of politicians, patients, staff and the public at large. To argue that managers do not practise in the domain of some form of rationality is to assume that they respond to pressures from different key stakeholders regardless of any moral principles.

Draper (1998) refers to the gulf which exists between the values of professional carers and those of managers. Some managers join the NHS from other industries and are usually on short-term contracts, typically for three years. They are often working on performance related pay where perform- ance is measured in terms of saving taxpayers' money.

> Thus, whilst they might for the duration of their contract adopt some of the values of health provision, this is a temporary adaptation to the industry in which their skills have been employed. . . . Ultimately, it is self-interest and professional pride in management skills which are the per- ceived sources of motivation.
>
> (Draper, 1998, p. 41)

Draper goes on to make an analogy between health care managers and politicians who might change portfolios and with industrial bosses who might be appointed to head a number of diverse enterprises in their management career. This happens, according to Draper, because management skills are readily transferable. The way to bridge the ethical gap between doctors and managers, says Draper, is to encourage and develop 'doctor-thinking managers' putting patients' interests as ends in themselves and not as possible means towards achieving waste reduction in certain areas of the organisation's activities. Alternatively, she argues, future health care managers should be trained within the NHS rather than being brought in from business and commerce with little knowledge of health care.

Draper's general statements about managers' ethical perspective are not presented with any foundation of empirical research findings. She ignores the fact that many trust and primary care organisation managers have been working within the NHS for many years and that clinicians have also been appointed to management posts. Furthermore, her regret at the gulf between professional carers' and managers' ethical stances is fuelled first by an assumption that professional ethics are of a higher order than management ethics, and second, by a further assumption that health care managers (in their role as managers, though they might also be clinicians) do not share or subscribe to the commitment to give the best possible service to each individual.

The contention that managers headhunted to go from one industry to another do not have a commitment to any particular business or industry (that they are merely applying skills to a different context) denies the possibility of transferring not just skills from one 'world' to another but also a transference of loyalty. She might just as well have cited the example of footballers who, having been transferred to another club, transfer only their skills and not their loyalty. The wish to work towards helping a club, business or NHS organisation thrive can involve the harnessing of individual self-interest (enjoying the job, gaining self-esteem and status, being rewarded financially) to the corporate mission.

Of course, it can be argued that the criteria for evaluating the 'success' of a football club or business are much clearer than those by which the NHS is assessed. Nevertheless, in any context the capacity of an organisation to achieve its primary, agreed aim will be its ability to attract and retain a sufficient number of highly skilled staff. Far from transferable skills being regarded, in Draper's view, as a deterrent to a *real* commitment to professional values, they offer an opportunity to assist highly complex health care organisations to meet the almost impossible task of achieving a multiplicity of objectives. The NHS is not a football club or a commercial enterprise. Utopian ideals have to be tempered with political and financial realities and in this endeavour, managers have an important contribution to make.

Summary

In this chapter we have tried to draw out the main political and ethical concepts that impinge upon decisions within the NHS. The values of different stakeholders are not easy to reconcile, particularly when changes have to be made in the balance of power between traditional and challenging groups.

The power of control over resources and where those resources should be distributed is the central issue in health care management, for this function operates at various levels. The difficult task of ensuring that the NHS remains true to its fundamental principle of equity of access to services is being tested by instances where 'postcode' prescribing appears to discriminate against people according to where they live. This inequitable situation leads to calls for more central control over resource allocation, and yet too much central control gives rise to accusations of authoritarianism. Politicians, therefore, have to combine direction with discretion.

In a similar fashion, health care managers need to balance their responsibility to the public with their accountability to political policy makers. There is still an unresolved tension between calls to empower patients and communities and the recognition of what that might mean in terms of resource allocation. While the central values that have guided the NHS over the decades are shared by the great majority of the public and by politicians and NHS workers, there is still, as we have argued here, a good deal of scope for differences and even conflicts to emerge in the management of health care services.

References

Alford, R. (1975) *Health Care Politics*. University of Chicago, Chicago.

Allison, G. (1971) *Essence of Decision*. Little Brown, Boston Mass.

Audit Commission (1986) *Making a Reality of Community Care*. HMSO, London.

Bachrach, P. & Baratz, M. (1962) 'Two faces of power'. *American Political Science Review*, **56**, pp. 641–51.

Baggott, R. (1998) *Health and Health Care in Britain*. Macmillan, London.

Brown, R. & Steel, D. (1979) *The Administrative Process in Britain*. Methuen, London.

Budge, I., Crewe, I., McKay, D. & Newton, K. (1998) *The New British Politics*. Addison Wesley Longman, Harlow.

Bulmer, M. (1982) *Social research ethics*. Macmillan, London.

Burch, M. & Wood, B. (1983) *Public Policy in Britain*. Martin Robertson, Oxford.

Chambers, D.E., Wedele, K. & Rodwell, M. (1992) *Evaluating social programs*. Allyn and Bacon, Boston, Mass.

Cheetham, J., Fuller, R., McIvor, G. & Petch, A. (1992) *Evaluating social work effectiveness*. Open University Press, Milton Keynes.

Coast, J., Donovan, J. & Frankl, S. (1996) *Priority Setting: the health care debate*. John Wiley, Chichester.

Dahl, R. (1957) 'The Concept of Power'. *Behavioural Science*, **2**, pp. 201–15.

Dahl, R. (1961) *Who Governs?* Yale University Press, New Haven, Conn.

Department of Health and Social Security (1989) *Working for Patients* (CM 555) HMSO, London.

Doyal, L. & Pennell, I. (1979) *The Political Economy of Health*. Pluto, London.

Draper, H. (1998) Should managers adopt the medical ethic? In: *Ethics and values in Health Care Management* (ed. Dracopolou, S.). Routledge, London.

Easton, D. (1965) *Framework for Political Analysis*. Prentice Hall, New Jersey.

Eckstein, H. (1960) *Pressure group politics*. Allen & Unwin, London.

Elcock, H. & Haywood, S. (1980) *The Buck Stops Where? Accountability and Control in the NHS*. University of Hull, Hull.

Enthoven, A. (1985) *Reflections on the Management of the NHS*. Nuffield Provincial Hospitals Trust, London.

Foucault, M. (1973) *The Birth of the Clinic*. Tavistock, London.

French, J. & Raven, B. (1968) The Bases of Social Power. In: *Group*

Dynamics: research and theory (eds Cartwright, D. & Zander, A.). Harper & Row, London.

Gillon, R. (1994) *Philosophical medical ethics*. John Wiley, New York.

Green, G.D. (2001) 'Philosophy for managers?' *Journal of Management in Medicine*, **15** (6), 488–98.

Griffiths, R. (1988) *Community Care: Agenda for Action*. HMSO, London.

Guardian, 10 June 2003.

Guba, E. & Lincoln, Y. (1989) *Fourth-Generation Evaluation*. Sage, Newbury Park.

Hailsham, Lord (1976) *Elective Dictatorship*. The Richard Dimbleby Lecture, BBC TV.

Ham, C. (1981) *Policy Making in the National Health Service*. Macmillan, London.

Ham, C. (1992) *Health Policy in Britain: the politics and organisation of the National Health Service*. Macmillan, London.

Handy, C. (1985) *Understanding organisations*. Penguin, Harmondsworth.

Harrison, S., Hunter, D. & Pollitt, C. (1990) *The Dynamics of British Health Policy*. Unwin Hyman, London.

Haywood, S. & Alaszewski, A. (1980) *Crisis in the Health Service: the politics of management*. Croom Helm, London.

Hill, M. (1997) *The Policy Process in the Modern State*. Prentice Hall/Harvester Wheatsheaf, London.

Hill, M. (1997) *The Policy Process: a Reader*. Prentice-Hall/Wheatsheaf, London.

Hogwood, B. & Gunn, L. (1984) *Policy analysis for the real world*. Oxford University Press, Oxford.

Hunter, F. (1953) *Community Power Structure*. University of North Carolina Press, Chapel Hill.

Illich, I. (1976) *Limits to Medicine*. Penguin, Harmondsworth.

Lee, K. & Mills, D. (1985) *Policy making and planning in the health sector*. Croom Helm, London.

Lindblom, C. (1959) 'The Science of "muddling through"'. *Public Administrative Review*, **19**, 78–88.

Loughlin, M. (1998) Impossible problems? In: *Ethics and Values in Health Care Management* (ed. Dracopolou, S.). Routledge, London.

Lukes, S. (1974) *Power: a Radical View*. Macmillan, London.

Macintyre, A. (1985) *After virtue: a study in moral theory*. Duckworth, London.

Maynard, A. (1991) 'Case for auditing audit?' *Health Service Journal*, 18 July, 26.

Navarro, V. (1978) *Class Struggle, the State and Medicine*. Martin Robertson, Oxford.

Nolan Committee (1995) *Standards in Public Life*. HMSO, London.

Ong, B., Boaden, M. & Cropper, S. (1997) 'Analysing the medicine-management interface in acute trusts'. *Journal of Management in Medicine*, **11** (2), 89–95.

Oregon Website (2003) www.ohd.hr.state.or.us

Palfrey, C. (2000) *Key concepts in health care policy and planning.* Macmillan, London.

Palfrey, C., Phillips, C., Thomas, P. & Edwards, D. (1992) *Policy Evaluation in the Public Sector*, Avebury, Aldershot.

Palfrey, C. & Thomas, P. (1996) 'Ethical issues in policy evaluation'. *Policy and Politics*, **24** (3), 277–86.

Palfrey, C. & Thomas, P. (1999) 'Politics and policy evaluation'. *Public Policy and Administration*, **14** (4), Winter, 58–70.

Palumbo, D. (1987) *The Politics of Program Evaluation.* Sage, Newbury Park.

Parker, M. (1998) *Ethics and Organisation.* Sage, London.

Punch, M. (1986) *The politics and ethics of fieldwork.* Sage, Beverley Hills, Calif.

Rhodes, R. & Dunleavy, P. (1995) *Prime Minister, Cabinet and Core Executive.* Macmillan, London.

Richardson, J. & Jordan, A. (1979) *Governing under Pressure.* Martin Robertson, Oxford.

Rist, R. (1995) *Policy Evaluation: linking theory to practice.* Edward Elgar, Aldershot.

Schattschneider, E. (1960) *The Semi-Sovereign People.* Holt, Rinehart and Winston, New York.

Sieber, J. (1980) Being ethical: professional and personal decisions in program evaluations. In: *Values, ethics and standards in evaluation* (eds Perloff, R. & Perloff, E.). Jolley Bass, San Francisco.

Smith, G. & Cantley, C. (1985) *Assessing Health Care: a study in organisational evaluation.* Open University, Milton Keynes.

Veney, J.E. & Kaluzny, A.D. (1984) *Evaluation and Decision Making for Health Services Programs.* Prentice Hall, New Jersey.

Wall, A. (1989) *Ethics and the health services manager.* King Edward's Hospital Fund for London, London.

Wall, A. (1994) 'Behind the wallpaper: a rejoinder'. *Health Care Analysis*, **2** (4), 317–18.

Weber, M. (1947) *The Theory of Social and Economic Organisation.* Oxford University Press, Oxford.

Williams, A. (1998) Economics, QALYs and medical ethics. In: *Ethics and Values in Health Care Management* (ed. Dracopolou, S.). Routledge, London.

Yukl, G. (1998) *Leadership in Organisations.* Prentice-Hall, New Jersey.

Chapter 7
Developing an Evaluative Approach to Health Care Management

Introduction

In Chapter 1 we outlined a model which we have found useful for analysing managerial and policy processes, especially processes involved in evaluation. Traditional systems approaches either ignore or under-emphasise the crucial elements of the model, which are the impact of incrementalism – particularly its political aspects – and the influence of value judgements. Conflicting perceptions, preferences and values are typical in debates about what ought to happen as far as health care policy and planning is concerned.

In terms of the 'outside boxes' of the model on page 4, there will commonly be differences of opinion concerning:

- the assessment of needs and problems
- priority setting in relation to goals and objectives
- the assessment of optional ways of achieving the objectives
- the processes by which policies and changes are implemented
- the evaluation of the outputs and outcomes of policies and services and the ways in which the results of evaluations are used

As far as evaluation processes are concerned, a key political question is who will decide:

- what data are to be collected?
- how the data will be collected and by whom?
- from whom data will be collected?
- what criteria will be used in coming to judgements about the policies and services being evaluated?
- how the criteria will be weighted?

- to what extent and in what ways the results of the evaluation will be fed back into the next phase of the policy making process?

All these are issues at the heart of contemporary health care management.

The past

Since the reorganisation of the NHS in 1974 the issue of management and, particularly in the early 1980s, the question of clinicians and management has been a recurring topic for discussion. Writing in 1981, Eskin (a practising GP) lamented the fact that 'medical training does not include a management component and in general doctors are not properly equipped to fulfil their management responsibilities' (Eskin, 1981, p. 3). She argues that the managerial role demands certain skills and is not a matter of mere common sense. Training for management, she asserts, should begin in the medical schools and continue into the postgraduate training period. She adds a comment relevant to current policy concerns, that: 'Those responsible for managing the service are more likely to feel a sense of commitment if they can be responsible for setting their own goals and objectives, even if this is constrained within the context of national policy' (p. 8).

Today, health care management is no longer a contestable concept as a function of both central government and devolved decision making. As far as a central role is concerned, since 1948 successive UK Governments have striven to implement, develop, curtail, contain and 'rationalise' the NHS. It has, in a cliché, become a victim of its own success. It has been a success not only in its preservation of an ideal – access to primary, secondary and tertiary health services largely free at the point of delivery – but in its contribution to enhanced life-saving treatments and a standard of care which continues to inspire public trust and confidence.

Dean (2003), for example, reported on the accolades bestowed on the unified NHS system by conference representatives from Australia, New Zealand and the USA. Overseas delegates singled out the following features of the NHS as particularly enviable developments: the creation of a national patient agency as the first stage towards the establishment of a national medical errors alert system; systematic assessment of new drugs and equipment; new national standards; the new General Medical Services contract and, above all, the new IT system that will link all parts of the NHS towards better integration of primary care and hospital services.

In an undertaking of this scale, it would be inconceivable that there would be no imperfections. The media regularly catalogues failures in reducing waiting lists and waiting times for operations and other health care interventions; medical errors; iatrogenic diseases and poor retention of nursing staff. Adverse events, which affect 5% of all patients admitted to hospitals in England and Wales, are known to cost the NHS about £500 million a year in additional days spent in hospital (Audit Commission, 2001) while adverse drug reactions in English hospitals cost £380 million per year, equivalent to 15–20 400-bed hospitals (Wiffen *et al.*, 2002). The cost of hospital acquired infection in England has been estimated at £930 million per annum, with infected patients staying in hospital for two weeks longer than those without infection (Plowman *et al.*, 2000).

Could all these negatives be the fault of managers or, perhaps, politicians – or both? Can these two sets of key players in the field of health care be responsible for any positive features of a still popular welfare service? What is the evidence for effective management having had any impact on the standard of health services and what is likely to be the position of managers in a future NHS?

Despite ideological antipathy to the stealthy intrusion of charges for prescriptions, for dental care and opthalmological services, politicians on the left have come to accept these compromises as no longer threatening the essential universality of a national health service. These are relatively minor erosions of a 'free' service. It is difficult for citizens of the UK who are not of a certain age to imagine the uncertainties, anxieties and fears of having to forego treatment because of an inability to meet the doctor's or hospital's fees.

One might regret the eventual exclusion from the 1911 National Insurance Act provisions of the obligatory contribution of the employer to the employee's health insurance payments and some might argue that this element should be restored.

Rising demand for health care is the reflection of a logic that might have escaped the vision of the original architects of the NHS. Certainly there was hope that universal access to treatments would, in time, improve the overall health of the nation to an extent that initial demand would taper off. Bevan, however, was not so sanguine and anticipated the need to increase resources (Hill, 1993). This almost passive assumption that 'free' or subsidised public services will inevitably lead to ever-increasing demand is, possibly, a tacit acknowledgement that state-run services are generally inefficient and wasteful of resources; that such a phenomenon is the unacceptable face of socialism. Certainly, it might appear to observers outside the UK that free consultations would lead to unnecessary visits to GPs and unwarranted demand on primary health care services.

In retrospect, it would appear that the bitter pill of managerialism has now proved to be an acceptable form of treatment for what was undeniably a public service in need of economic rehabilitation. Pumping more and more money into the NHS has proved to be no remedy for the health care dilemma depicted in Chapter 5. Perhaps there was a need for more radical, lateral thinking. One response to this virtually universal problem in health care provision is to dampen demand. The means to achieve this can be varied. For example, the free market economy of the USA places the responsibility for health care firmly on the individual. But for those unable to provide for the health care needs of themselves and family through insurance mechanisms, the scenario is a pre-NHS situation in the UK: the economically disadvantaged become excluded from the system.

In Singapore, the highly centralist Government has adopted a different strategy for containing spiralling demands on Government health care budgets. Recognising that supply is likely to stimulate demand, the Government has implemented a policy to restrict subsidised health services to a basic level of care and treatment, particularly with respect to hospital environment and amenities, and placed a cap on the numbers of doctors to be trained. The logic in the Government's policy document of 1992 ('Affordable Health Care', Ministry of Health, 1992), which is still the current policy, is that by containing the numbers of doctors who might work in the private sector, this will reduce public expectations about what services could and should be provided through Government subsidies.

This policy initiative, to dampen demand or to 'de-market', has never overtly been attempted in Britain. The 'management' of the health service has traditionally been characterised by an uneasy compromise between implicit rationing through waiting lists and the introduction of charges which has neither added significantly to the NHS budget nor deterred the public from unnecessarily visiting the GP. Repugnant as it has been to many idealists wedded to the preservation of a national health service rooted in the aftermath of World War II, with all the national aspirations for a more equitable society, the introduction of a more hardnosed approach to demand and resources has tended to be misconstrued as the implementation of a political ideology alien to the concept of an inclusive health service. Against this response to the reforms and innovations in the 1980s, an argument could be put forward that presents these reforms not as an assault upon the very concept of a nationalised health care industry, but a genuine attempt to ensure that the NHS survived through the medium of good management.

The present

In the context of public services in Britain, we live in an increasingly evaluative culture. This assertion would seem to fit well with the argument developed in this book that health care management needs to embed a reflective appraisal approach into all organisational activities. However, we have also maintained that the process of evaluation necessarily involves *a priori* value positions and pragmatic political concerns. In an enterprise as huge and as complex as the NHS, there are a variety of constituents or stakeholders to accommodate. Therefore, at all levels of governance, political adroitness is a key competence in sailing between the Scylla and Charybdis of professional interests and public expectations.

Part of the legacy of early resistance to the influx of non-clinically trained managers into the NHS still appears to dog the public image of managers. Preston and Loan-Clarke (2000) reported that NHS managers were very aware of the largely negative perceptions that surround them but accept that this is an integral part of the job. Wall also noted that 'the most uncomfortable position in the managerial hierarchy' was that of the middle manager (Wall, 1999, p. 22). Perhaps we have moved some way from the sturdily sceptical view expressed by Pollitt in his definition of 'managerialism': 'A set of beliefs and practices at the core of which burns the seldom-tested assumption that better management will provide an effective solvent for a wide range of economic ills' (Pollitt, 1990, p. 1).

Yet the dichotomy between 'managers' and 'professionals' as distinct interest groups within the NHS is probably still intact. If so, this is unfortunate because it tacitly denotes a lower status to managers and denies the possibility of their becoming accepted as professionals in their own right. Perhaps the absence of any recognised educational career or qualification, other than perhaps the MBA, militates against NHS managers being accepted as having specialist knowledge and skills. Several courses at Masters level exist in British universities but these are usually designed for people already in posts in health care from the UK and overseas and not as preparatory to entering the service. Action to assure professional management development is being taken by the NHS Confederation which, in 2003, stated its objective to explore the role of chief executives and NHS boards and the changes needed to support management excellence (NHS Confederation, 2003). And in the same year, the Centre for Health Leadership in Wales set out its intention to develop an accredited continuing professional development programme (CPD) framework for NHS managers which will adopt the

Institute of Health Care Management 'Code of Conduct' (Health Professions, Wales, 2003).

While these initiatives to improve standards of management are well intentioned, they are somewhat limited in their scope. What we are proposing is that managers need to acquire knowledge of and competence in a variety of evaluation methods and designs in order to encourage and sustain an evaluative culture at primary care and NHS trust level and that by doing so, they will be exerting much needed leadership in the area of clinical governance. More broadly, the ability of managers to respond to apparently inconsistent and conflicting demands regarding what and how to evaluate is undoubtedly a competence of considerable importance as far as risk management is concerned.

While we acknowledge that an evaluative culture is ostensibly a positive policy generated by successive Governments over the past 20 years, confusion and some hostility can arise when there is disagreement 'from below' about the nature of the evaluation. In 2003, the outgoing chairman of the British Medical Association complained about a health care system 'driven by spreadsheets and tick boxes' (*The Times*, 1 July). Dr Ian Bogle said that a target-driven Government had created a climate of fear and deception that distorted medical practice and forced the honest to lie. Delegates at the BMA meeting addressed by Dr Bogle expressed their dissatisfaction with targets, star ratings and the prospect of foundation hospitals. The chairman accused the Government of eroding clinical freedom and turning the NHS into 'the most centralised public service in the free world'.

He went on to talk of 'production-line values' which produce nationally set targets without any appreciation of what they might mean for doctors in consulting rooms with individual patients. Interestingly, the outgoing chairman did not see managers as handmaidens of the Government but expressed sympathy for the lengths to which NHS managers were compelled to go in order to satisfy ministers. Strategies included manipulation of waiting lists, keeping patients in ambulances so that Accident and Emergency targets could be met, and classifying patients as admitted to hospital even though they were still on trolleys. For this public indictment of Government policy Dr Bogle was given a standing ovation. However, this politically driven concern, if not passion, for imposing standards or targets to be used as indicators of quality performance is driven by a very worthy attempt to make public services and public servants more accountable to the Government and to the taxpayer.

While the delegates from overseas at the conference reported by Dean (2003) referred with acclaim to the 'unified system' in Britain compared, for example, with the multiple provider and complex arrangement of federal subsidies operative in the USA, a unified system can become a 'centralist autocracy' in the view of health care professionals. Yet, it could be argued that, in Britain, the idea of a unified system relates only to the NHS and not to the wider health and health care environment in which private provision is available as, of course, it has been since the inception of the NHS. The reason that the ex-chairman of the BMA received a standing ovation from his peers was probably because of a gap between expectation and reality. The delegation of service purchasing and provision decisions to trust level has not brought with it enhanced discretion with regard to prioritising which services should be supplied. To many in the NHS, health care management is really done at central government level. What is delegated to primary and secondary care levels might seem more like the administration of ministerial decisions.

The future

There are, however, some indications of change in the balance between centrally imposed standards and local autonomy. The new 'localism' identified by Walker (2003) is a recognition by certain Government ministers that excessively detailed targets are dysfunctional. According to Walker's sources, Whitehall promises fewer targets and much less 'pseudo-quantification'. The case for foundation hospital trusts was planned (for the autumn of 2003) to emphasise their democratic legitimacy based on patients and citizens voting in the governing boards. Elsewhere, in the British public sector, local authorities will no longer need to present so many detailed plans for Whitehall approval and the better councils will receive fewer inspections. Walker, however, is not convinced that this apparent move towards more locally centred decision making will be sustained. He argues:

> Intellectually the Treasury may now accept that corset-tight quantitative targets do have perverse effects, focusing managers' attention on meeting them rather than public service at large. But, practically, the keepers of the public purse are going to insist no less rigorously than before that councils – and health trusts – prove they are worth it.
>
> (Walker, 2003, p. 14)

The other source of an impetus for change in the central-local relationship is the Wanless Report (2002) and the Review of Health and Social Care in Wales (Welsh Assembly Government, 2003) in which Derek Wanless acted as an adviser to the Welsh Assembly Government. In both documents the importance of engaging with the public in decision making is stressed, and while standards should continue to be set centrally, the principle of local solutions to local issues must be adopted and the relationship between national roles and local freedoms needs to be clarified.

There are signs that the present Government at the beginning of the twenty-first century is keen to move away from what it regards as outdated dogma and towards an era of eclectic politics. No longer wedded to the ideology of socialism, it has sought to distance itself from any ism, preferring to countenance a number of options towards achieving particular ends. According to this political agenda, the commitment to a health service largely free at the point of delivery is still intact but if services can be provided at less cost to the Government and at less inconvenience, if laundry and catering services can be turned over to private companies, what could be more logical than to franchise the management of key NHS organisations to the private sector?

At the time of writing (the summer of 2003), the post of chief executive in an NHS trust in the Midlands in England was to be filled by a person or management team employed by a private sector firm. In some respects, therefore, trusts do enjoy degrees of autonomy, provided that the decision to engage with the private sector is done in the name of efficiency as defined by central Government (Shifrin, 2003).

Bearing in mind successive exhortations in policy documents for more meaningful public and patient participation within the health care system, it remains to be seen whether real participation and consultation by trusts will happen. By 'real' we mean much more than tokenisim – that is, consultation in the form of a public relations exercise. Real participation would come close to equal partnership in decision making. To work properly as far as this degree of public involvement is concerned, it would be inadequate to reproduce at more micro level the form of representative democracy that characterises decision making from Westminster or the devolved institutions in Northern Ireland, Scotland and Wales. Particularly at primary care level, the responsibility to interact with the local communities is a policy imperative that could conceivably lead to distinctive local prioritising that sits uncomfortably with or seriously challenges centrally determined targets and objectives.

This possibility would mean the politicising of health care planning and more so when local authorities, working closely with primary care organisations, are not of the same political persuasion as the current Government. In this scenario, the challenge for health care management will be profound. For, contrary to the argument of some commentators quoted in Chapter 6, who view health care managers as resembling unreflecting bureaucrats, our position is that the model of decision making presented in Chapter 1 is more in line with reality than a mechanistic rational model that gives little or no prominence to the key influence of values.

Summary

Evaluation is, in essence, ascribing values to observed processes, outputs and outcomes. Management is more than control and the implementation of correct procedures. It must surely be about leadership and creativity where values guide both policy and practice. Assessing the needs of local communities and responding to those needs has to have regard to matters relating to equity, empathy and equality as well as economy, efficiency and effectiveness. In the near future, health care managers might be encouraged by the results of truly participative decision making as a counter to centrally determined targets, in order to work with an alliance of local authorities and voluntary organisations to identify the criteria by which local health services will be evaluated. The really effective health care manager will combine a continuous self-evaluation through performance measurement 'from below' as well as 'from above' with a capacity to monitor, appraise and assess the success of the organisation from the perspective of all stakeholders.

References

Audit Commission (2001) *A spoonful of sugar: medicines management in NHS hospitals*. Audit Commission, London.

Dean, M. (2003) 'The oldest and still the best'. *Guardian Society*, 16 July, 7.

Eskin, F. (1981) *Doctors and Management Skills*. MCB Publications, Bradford.

Health Professions Wales (2003) 'Pathways to performance: developing clinical leadership in Wales'. *Newyddion*, March, 6.

Hill, M. (1993) *The Welfare State in Britain*. Edward Elgar, Aldershot.

Ministry of Health (1992) *Affordable health care for all: executive summary*. Ministry of Health, Singapore.

NHS Confederation (2003) *Working for Primary Care Trusts*. NHS Confederation, London.

Plowman, R., Graves, N., Griffin, M., Roberts, J.A., Swan, A.V., Cookson, B.D. & Taylor, L. (2000) *Socio-economic burden of hospital acquired infection*. Public Health Laboratory Service, London.

Pollitt, C. (1990) *Managerialism and the Public Sector*. Blackwell, Oxford.

Preston, D. & Loan-Clarke, J. (2000) 'The NHS manager: a view from the bridge'. *Journal of Management in Medicine*, **14** (2), 100–108.

Shifrin, T. (2003) 'Out on a limb'. *Guardian Society*, 4 June, 13.

The Times (2003) 'BMA head attacks "cheating on figures"'. 1 July, 2.

Walker, D. (2003) 'All at sea'. *Guardian Society*, 30 July, 14.

Wall, A. (1999) 'Courtin' the middle'. *Health Service Journal* (109) 4 Feb, 22–5.

Wanless Report (2002) *Securing our Future Health: taking a long-term view*. Department of Health, London.

Welsh Assembly Government (2003) *Review of Health and Social Care in Wales*. WAG, Cardiff.

Wiffen, P., Gill, M., Edwards, J. & Moore, A. (2002) 'Adverse drug reactions in hospital patients: a systematic review of the prospective and retrospective studies'. http://www.jr2.ox.ac.uk/bandolier/Extraforbando/ADRPM.pdf

Index